A PRACTICAL GUIDE TO
Assessing the Competency of Low-Volume Providers

HUGH GREELEY

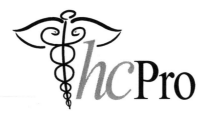

A *Practical Guide to Assessing the Competency of Low-Volume Providers* is published by HCPro, Inc.

HCPro provides information resources for the healthcare industry. A selected listing of our products is listed in the back of this book.

HCPro is not affiliated in any way with the Joint Commission on Accreditation of Healthcare Organizations, which owns the JCAHO trademark.

Hugh Greeley, Author
Erin E. Callahan, Senior Managing Editor
Dale Seamans, Executive Editor
Jean St. Pierre, Creative Director
Mike Mirabello, Senior Graphic Artist
Susan Darbyshire, Layout Artist
Tom Philbrook, Cover Designer
Kathyrn Levesque, Group Publisher
Suzanne Perney, Publisher

Advice given is general. Readers should consult professional counsel for specific legal, ethical, or clinical questions. Arrangements can be made for quantity discounts.

For more information on this or any other HCPro publication, contact:
HCPro
P.O. Box 1168
Marblehead, MA 01945
Telephone: 800/650-6787 or 781/639-1872
Fax: 781/639-2982
E-mail: *customerservice@hcpro.com*

Visit HCPro at its World Wide Web sites:
www.hcpro.com, www.hcmarketplace.com

08/2004
20086

CONTENTS

CONTENTS

About the Author

Hugh P. Greeley

Hugh P. Greeley is the founder of The Greeley Company, a division of HCPro, Inc. Mr. Greeley has participated as a faculty member in over 2,500 seminars on the subjects of medical staff organization, quality improvement, credentialing, trustee responsibility, antitrust, accreditation, and other related subjects. Mr. Greeley was a member of the board and professional affairs committee of Deaconess-Incarnate Word Health System in St. Louis. In addition, he was one of the founding partners of The Credentialing Institute and a contributing editor to many healthcare journals. Mr. Greeley has also been a member of the Estes Park Institute and the American College of Physician Executives.

Mr. Greeley is also the chair of the board of the Volunteers In Medicine Institute, a not-for-profit organization dedicated to assisting medical staffs, hospitals, and communities in the development of clinics serving the uninsured.

Prior to founding The Greeley Company, Mr. Greeley held a number of positions with the Joint Commission on Accreditation of Healthcare Organizations, InterQual, Inc., and Kenosha Hospital Medical Center. He is also the author of numerous publications and articles.

INTRODUCTION

How to use this book

In hospitals across the country, medical services professionals (MSPs), department chairs, credentials committee members, and medical executive committee (MEC) members increasingly face requests for medical staff membership, reappointment, and clinical privileges submitted by physicians with little or no clinical volume. Such physicians are commonly referred to as low- and no-volume practitioners.

Hospitals must adopt new strategies for responding to physicians' decisions to rely less on the hospital for care and treatment of patients. Unfortunately, in many instances, the medical staff's current bylaws, ingrained practices, and fear of the unknown may prevent the hospital from taking a common-sense approach to an appointment or privileging request submitted by a low- or no-volume practitioner. This book will teach medical staff and credentialing professionals how to process such requests.

Issue: Physicians who traditionally have little call for hospital resources—allergists, dermatologists, dentists, etc.—are now increasingly joined by family physicians, internists, surgeons, pediatricians, and other physicians with active office practices. These physicians are choosing to limit their hospital practices and instead refer acutely ill patients to hospitalists and other hospital physicians for inpatient care. This trend means that hospital credentialing professionals have limited access to competency data on which to base medical staff appointment and clinical privilege decisions that affect these practitioners.

Turn to existing policies

For many hospitals, the answers to the questions posed by low- and no-volume providers can be found in the organization's current policies, procedures, and bylaws. Traditional medical staff bylaws often prevent credentialing and medical staff professionals from effectively processing such providers' medical staff membership requests by requiring that practitioners on the active medical staff perform a large number of procedures at the facility.

This book will help you analyze your current bylaws and amend them to allow your organization to effectively address membership and privileging requests made by the increasing number of low- and no-volume physicians in your community.

How to gather competency data

A Practical Guide to Assessing the Competency of Low-Volume Providers will teach you how to apply basic credentialing rules to physicians who have no or minimal volume at your hospital.

For example, many low- and no-volume physicians provide clinical services at another accredited inpatient or ambulatory facility. Experienced medical services procession-als, department chairs, and credentials committee members already know how to process applications submitted by such providers. After all, your organization processes an application from a provider with no clinical volume at your hospital every time it receives a new application for medical staff membership.

When processing such initial medical staff applications, the medical staff and governing board rely primarily on evidence gathered from the facility that attests to the applicant's clinical activity and quality of care. Therefore, reappointment or clinical privileging request submitted by a current medical staff member who chooses to perform most or all of his or her work at another facility should not pose significant problems for your hospital's credentialing professionals as long as you gather adequate references and information attesting to the physician's practice quality and volume from the other facility. However, the physician's decision to practice primarily at another facility may affect his or her staff category at your hospital.

This book will show that responding to a request for continued clinical privileges from a physician who performs all or most of his or her work at another facility is not primarily a clinical issue, but rather a patient safety issue that you can successfully address by developing new policies and thoughtfully applying current policies.

A *Practical Guide to Assessing the Competency of Low-Volume Providers* also aims to teach your hospital that it has options—beyond outright denial of medical staff membership or clinical privileges—when responding to an application submitted by a low- or no-volume provider. This book will prepare your organization's medical staff and credentialing team to react confidently when it is next faced with such a request.

Chapter by chapter

To address the challenges presented by physicians who do not need to use the hospital's resources regularly, you must understand the terms that are typically used when discussing this issue. Toward this end, we've included a glossary in the following section of the book.

Chapter one provides insight into low- and no-volume physicians by offering examples of providers that fit this definition and by explaining why they are a growing challenge.

Chapter two gives a complete overview of the appraisal/reappraisal process. This overview provides you a solid foundation that will allow your organization to decide how it will process medical staff membership and clinical privileges requests submitted by low- and no-volume providers. Chapter two also includes an algorithm to clarify each step of the process and to detail your options as you progress through the appraisal/reappraisal process.

Chapter three takes the lessons you learned in the previous chapters and explains how to apply them to low- and no-volume providers.

Chapter four discusses options for responding to medical staff membership and privileging requests made by low- and no-volume practitioners, and shows you how the details of individual cases affect those options. This chapter also explains the importance of separating the issue of medical staff membership from that of clinical privileges. Although both appointment to the medical staff and granting of clinical privileges are part of the credentialing process, the two are not one in the same.

This chapter also addresses the importance of ensuring that your medical staff policies and procedures allow your organization to properly respond when faced with an application submitted by a low- or no-volume provider. This chapter presents a typical scenario and then discusses how the process for responding to that scenario is affected by different low- and no-volume providers.

Chapter five includes three hypothetical case studies involving appraisal and reappraisal challenges that all hospital credentialing professionals are likely to face. After presenting the details surrounding the submission of a medical staff membership application or clinical privilege request by a low- or no-volume provider, we present strategies for responding appropriately to the request. These case studies will prepare your hospital to address similar situations confidently.

To help your organization implement our recommendations, we have provided throughout the book practical forms and tools, including reference questionnaires, sample policies and letters, an intended practice plan, and the new credentialing standard.

GLOSSARY

The following list of terms will help you better follow the discussion of low- and no-volume providers in this book and prepare you to address the challenges presented by these providers at your organization.

- **The competency equation** is a simple approach to the information your credentials committee, department chair, medical executive committee, and governing board need to grant clinical privileges appropriately.

  To fulfill the competency equation, you must gather evidence of actual performance (relating to the practitioner's request for clinical privilege) and evidence of the quality of that performance. This information helps your organization determine whether the practitioner is currently clinically competent to perform the requested clinical privileges.

  However, performance alone is not sufficient to determine competency.

  Similarly, letters, completed questionnaires, and reports submitted by the practitioner's department chair that attest to his or her competence do not provide complete information. These letters may attest to the physician's past clinical competence, but they do not provide information about recent clinical activity.

  Therefore, the competency equation requires you to gather both evidence of actual performance and evidence of outcomes to determine a practitioner's current clinical competence.

- **Current clinical competence** is a term used by the Joint Commission on Accreditation of Healthcare Organizations to refer to the parameters a practitioner must meet to be granted clinical privileges. "Current" refers to a recent time period.

"Clinical" refers to the requested privileges. "Competence" refers to evidence that the physician's past performance of the requested privileges met the organization's standards for quality in regard to skill, judgment, and overall performance.

When requesting clinical privileges, a practitioner must provide the hospital with evidence that he or she has the training and experience necessary to competently carry out the requested privileges. That is, he or she must demonstrate current clinical competence.

- **Dependent privileges** authorize a physician to provide clinical services only in conjunction with, or under the direct supervision of, a qualified practitioner.

- **Equivalency** comes into play when processing a medical staff membership application submitted by a low- or no-volume provider. In such situations, a medical staff may choose to rely on evidence of the practitioner's continuing medical education or reasonably comparable ambulatory practice in the absence of inpatient practice data.

- **Independent privileges** allow a practitioner to care for patients independently of other qualified practitioners. A physician is most often granted independent privileges, which allow him or her to treat patients without consulting or getting the approval of another caregiver.

- **Low- and no-volume practitioners** perform few or no procedures at the hospital. A low- and no-volume practitioner has a clinical volume at your facility that is lower than that specified by the minimum threshold criteria for clinical privilege, as established by your medical staff.

These physicians may rely on your organization's hospitalist program, refer the majority of their patients to another facility for inpatient care, or focus on their office practices. Whatever the reason for their absence from your hospital, the challenge they present to your medical services and credentialing team is the same: the absence of clinical data makes it difficult to verify their competence.

- **Medical staff appointment** allows physicians access to the physicians' dining room, hospital library, continuing medical education classes, and voting rights if allowed by hospital policy. In addition, medical staff membership allows the physician to advertise his or her affiliation with your organization and to satisfy managed care organizations' requirements.

The hospital's board makes the final decision whether to grant or deny an application for medical staff appointment. To make this decision, the board reviews the physician's application, a summary of pertinent information, the department chair's recommendation, the credentials committee's recommendation (when applicable), the medical executive committee's (MEC's) recommendations, and any applicable guidelines or rules.

It's important that your credentials committee and MEC recommend membership criteria to the governing board before applying them to a medical staff applicant. Once the board approves the criteria, write them into the medical staff bylaws and policies.

Upon appointment, the practitioner must apply for permission to treat specific conditions and perform specific procedures. Remember, the term "credentialing" refers to the overall process of gathering and verifying credentials information, reviewing that information, and making a decision to grant or deny medical staff membership. Although both appointment to the medical staff and granting of clinical privileges are part of the credentialing process, they are not one and the same. See Chapter four for more information.

In addition to deciding whether to grant an applicant medical staff appointment, the board must determine to which staff category to appoint the applicant. This decision depends on the practitioner's interest in meeting the institutions' mission.

Lastly, the board may also decide to which department to appoint the applicant, which is generally based on the practitioner's training and area of practice.

- **Medical staff responsibilities** are generally defined in the medical staff bylaws. The bylaws should clearly state the practitioner's responsibilities as a member of the medical staff, taking into account the physician's staff category and department appointment. An increasing number of medical staffs require all members to accept responsibility for emergency department coverage, committee assignment, peer review, and performance improvement.

- **Privileges** are the procedures that the hospital permits the practitioner to perform. Determining the procedures that each medical staff appointee may perform and conditions that he or she may treat—commonly known as "delineation of privileges"—is one of the most difficult jobs that department chairs and other medical staff leaders face.

  The delineation of clinical privileges requires fair and consistent analysis of each appointee's education, training, experience, and clinical competence to determine whether they match the particular procedures that the appointee wishes to perform.

- **Staff prerogatives** are generally defined in the medical staff bylaws. They state with extreme clarity the prerogatives associated with appointment, category, or departmental assignment. These prerogatives generally include voting and holding a medical staff office.

• **Threshold criteria** for requesting privileges refers to the minimum education, training, and experience an applicant or reapplicant must have to qualify for independent clinical privileges. Physicians must meet this threshold before the medical staff office will process their application or reapplication. For example, a physician who seeks privileges to admit and treat patients must successfully complete an approved residency training program in either family or internal medicine. Candidates must also demonstrate provision of inpatient care, as the primary attending physician, to at least 10 patients during the past year.

THE INCREASE OF LOW- AND NO-VOLUME PROVIDERS

Your credentials committee likely has had a reappointment request before them in the past year that was submitted by a physician who admitted few or no patients to your facility during his or her soon-to-be expired appointment period.

The credentials committee also likely received a medical staff application/clinical privilege request from a physician who has not provided inpatient care for many years, admits all of his or her patients to another hospital in the community, or works exclusively in his or her office.

Yours is not the only credentials committee confronted with the challenge of processing such appointment requests.

Medical services professionals, department chairs, and credentials committee members in hospitals across the country are faced increasingly with applications for medical staff membership or clinical privileges from physicians who treat few or no patients at their hospital.

Hospitals and credentialing professionals, understandably, are concerned about this trend and its effect on the credentialing process. These concerns are elevated by fear that the hospital will not meet accreditation standards and fear that a physician may lack the skills and knowledge to care appropriately for patients. In addition, hospitals worry that a low- or no-volume physician may admit and treat a patient who subsequently files a corporate negligence suit against the hospital, accusing the hospital of negligent retention.

The emergence of low- and no-volume providers

There are many explanations for a decline in a physician's activity at the hospital—he or she may have relied on your organization's hospitalist program, referred a majority of his or her patients to another facility for inpatient care, or focused attention on his or her office practice.

LOW-VOLUME AND NO-VOLUME PROVIDERS USUALLY FALL INTO THE FOLLOWING THREE CATEGORIES:

1. The provider treats the majority or all of his or her patients at another inpatient facility

2. The physician is not clinically active at another inpatient facility but is active within the community (e.g., family physician, dermatologist, or allergist)

3. The physician has not practiced medicine for several years

---

Whatever the reason for the decline in hospital activity, processing medical staff applications and privileging requests from such providers have many credentialing and medical staff professionals stumped. And the biggest stumbling block is the absence of data with which to assess the physician's competence.

Remember, competency is the main issue during appointment, reappointment, and privileging, whether the physician is an active member of the medical staff or is a low- or no-volume provider.

Absence of competency data

The phenomenon of low- and no-volume providers is relatively new and has arisen primarily because of general internists' and family physicians' decision to change the way they practice medicine. That is, more and more of these practitioners are finding it beneficial to devote time to their office-based practices rather than providing inpatient services.

It's not difficult to understand why these physicians are concentrating on their office-based practices. However, physicians' decisions to do so make reappointment an even more difficult task as medical staff and credentialing professionals struggle to gather competency data for physicians with limited or no hospital activity.

In Chapter three, we will present strategies to help your organization gather the competency data it needs to confidently appoint a low- or no-volume practitioner to its medical staff.

UNDERSTAND THE APPRAISAL AND REAPPRAISAL PROCESS

You must understand each step of the medical staff appraisal/reappraisal process before you can effectively tackle the challenges presented by low- and no-volume providers' medical staff appointment and reappointment requests. A firm understanding of this process will help you decide what steps your organization will take to process a membership/clinical privilege request submitted by a physician who has little or no clinical activity at your facility.

Let's begin this discussion by looking at a complete algorithm detailing the reappointment process. Turn to **Figure 2.0** on p. 6. This chapter will walk you through each step of the process depicted on the flowchart.

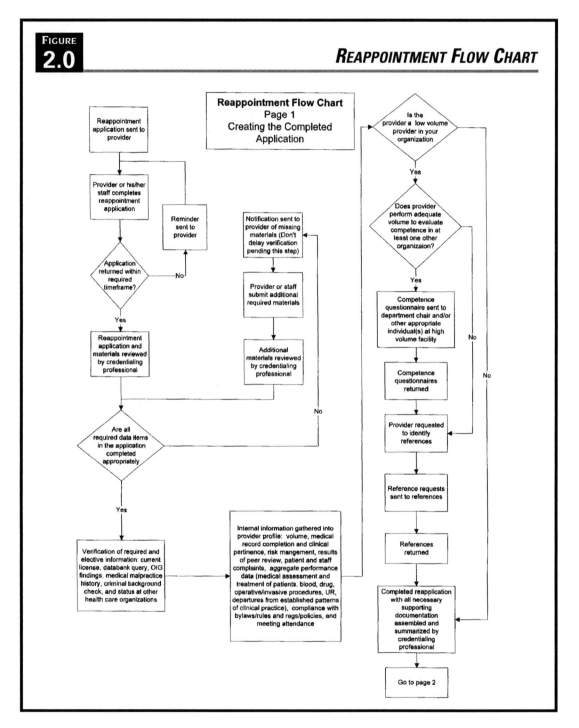

FIGURE 2.0

REAPPOINTMENT FLOW CHART

Reappointment Flow Chart
Page 1
Creating the Completed
Application

Reappointment application sent to provider

Provider or his/her staff completes reappointment application

Application returned within required timeframe?

No

Reminder sent to provider

Yes

Reappointment application and materials reviewed by credentialing professional

Are all required data items in the application completed appropriately

Yes

No

Verification of required and elective information: current license, databank query, OIG findings, medical malpractice history, criminal background check, and status at other health care organizations

Notification sent to provider of missing materials (Don't delay verification pending this step)

Provider or staff submit additional required materials

Additional materials reviewed by credentialing professional

No

Internal information gathered into provider profile: volume, medical record completion and clinical pertinence, risk mangement, results of peer review, patient and staff complaints, aggregate performance data (medical assessment and treatment of patients, blood, drug, operative/invasive procedures, UR, departures from established patterns of clinical practice), compliance with bylaws/rules and regs/policies, and meeting attendance

Is the provider a low volume provider in your organization

Yes

Does provider perform adequate volume to evaluate competence in at least one other organizaion?

Yes

No

Competence questionnaire sent to department chair and/or other appropriate individual(s) at high volume facility

No

Competence questionnaires returned

Provider requested to identify references

Reference requests sent to references

References returned

Completed reapplication with all necessary supporting documentation assembled and summarized by credentialing professional

Go to page 2

FIGURE 2.0

REAPPOINTMENT FLOW CHART (CONT.)

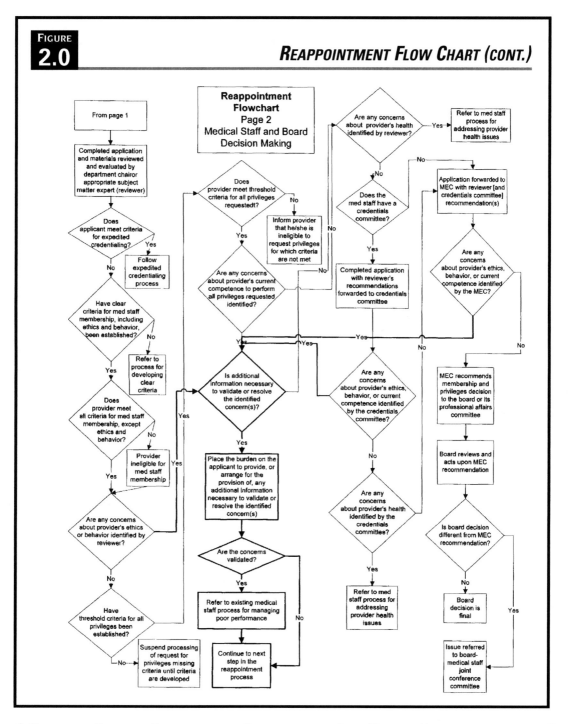

Appraisal and reappraisal: Step by step

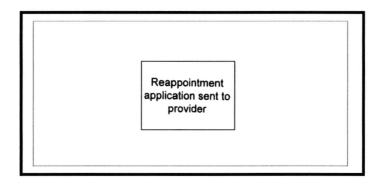

Reappointment
application sent to
provider

Step one: In nearly every hospital in the United States, the appraisal and reappraisal process begins with the completion of a formal application or reapplication. See **Figure 2.1** on p. 30 for a sample application for medical staff appointment and clinical privileges.

The completed application should provide the hospital with important information about the physician applicant's education, training, and experience. When reviewing your current medical staff application to ensure that it collects all necessary information, read through the applicable standards from the Joint Commission on Accreditation of Healthcare Organizations or the Health Care Facilities Accreditation program. In addition, take a look at **Figure 2.2** on p. 38 for information about the evolving credentialing standard.

In addition to the formal application, many hospitals require that the practitioner provide information in support of his or her application. For example, some medical staff offices (MSOs) require the physician to submit copies of licenses, diplomas, and residency completion letters as part of the application process.

Although it is perfectly acceptable to require this information, doing so adds to the overall bureaucracy of the application and reapplication process. It does not add significant value because all information directly submitted to the MSO by the practitioner must be verified by primary or acceptable secondary sources.

Note: MSOs typically require this information as a result of past difficulty verifying physicians' background and training. The requirement was more valuable when it was more difficult to forge complicated certificates. However, widely available technology, such as scanners and photocopiers, make it possible to fabricate any document. Therefore, only primary or equivalent secondary-source verification can prevent such falsification.

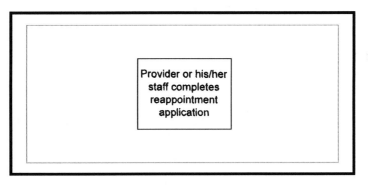

Provider or his/her staff completes reappointment application

Step two: When the practitioner receives the application or reapplication from the hospital, he or she must ensure that all forms are completed and returned to the MSO.

With the application, the hospital should include instructions that specify whether the material must be hand-printed or typed. Additionally, instructions should indicate that the hospital will consider the application void if it is not returned within a designated timeframe.

See **Figure 2.3** on p. 43 for sample instructions on how to complete the application for medical staff appointment.

In addition to the traditional paper application, more and more MSOs are using online application and reapplication forms. A few organizations now send a hospital designee to meet with physicians and assist them in completing the application.

Regardless of which mechanism your facility chooses, the entire process should be halted if the practitioner does not return the completed application or reapplication form—along with all required additional material—to the MSO within the specified timeframe.

Tip: Take steps to ensure that a physician's failure to return or satisfactorily complete application or reapplication forms does not result in significant work for the medical services professional (MSP). To do so, the MSO should develop a simple checklist that can be sent to all practitioners who fail to return necessary documents. The checklist should indicate the information the practitioner applicant must complete and return to the hospital. See **Figure 2.4** on p. 46 for a sample application completion checklist. The checklist should also state that if the applicant does not provide the required information within a designated timeframe, the MSO will terminate the application process and take no further action. Including this statement means that the MSO is not required to take action if the applicant fails to respond to the notice.

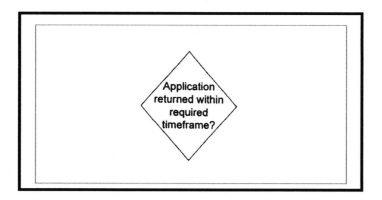

Step three: The MSP must determine whether the practitioner has completed the application or reapplication form appropriately and returned it to the MSO within the required timeframe.

If the practitioner fails to complete the documents, the hospital may send the physician a reminder to encourage him or her to return the form. See **Figure 2.5** on p. 49 for a sample notification of failure to submit application.

Note: MSPs use innovative techniques to ensure that practitioner applicants promptly return forms to the hospital. Even with these techniques, however, many hospitals are forced to send reminder notices and otherwise encourage the practitioner to complete the form prior to expiration of their appointment.

MSPs who experiment with new techniques report that a fairly straightforward letter, which indicates that the MSO will issue a monetary fine if the physician submits the application after a certain date, works very well. This letter should accompany the medical staff appointment application and should note that the MSO will not process the application of a physician who fails to pay this fine.

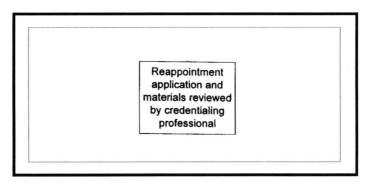

Reappointment
application and
materials reviewed
by credentialing
professional

Step four: Once the applicant or reapplicant has submitted his or her forms, the MSP or an appropriate assistant must carefully review the documents.

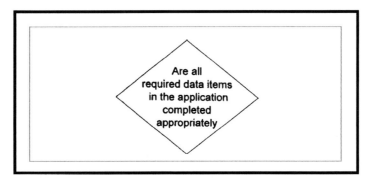

Are all
required data items
in the application
completed
appropriately

Step five: If upon review of the practitioner's completed application the MSP determines that the applicant did not return all requested materials, the MSP should notify the physician of the omission. The notification letter should make it clear that the practitioner must submit the required information by a specified date.

While waiting for the additional materials, the MSP should verify the information on the application. If the practitioner does return the additional documents, the MSP must review that information to determine whether the application is now complete.

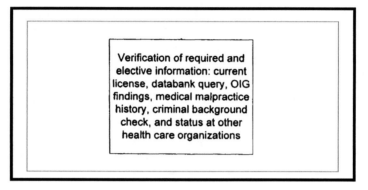

Verification of required and elective information: current license, databank query, OIG findings, medical malpractice history, criminal background check, and status at other health care organizations

Step six: When the MSO determines that the application is complete, the MSP or credentials committee must then verify the information on it. This step can be accelerated with the assistance of the Internet. Nearly all the information needed to verify education, training, licensure status, board status, certain prior disciplinary actions, governmental sanctions, and "successful" malpractice actions can be obtained using the Internet. However, some information on the application must be verified by a phone, fax, or letter.

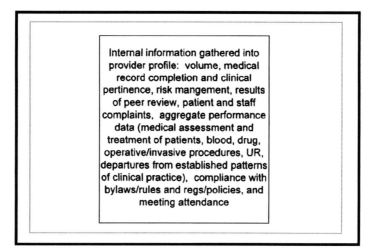

Internal information gathered into provider profile: volume, medical record completion and clinical pertinence, risk mangement, results of peer review, patient and staff complaints, aggregate performance data (medical assessment and treatment of patients, blood, drug, operative/invasive procedures, UR, departures from established patterns of clinical practice), compliance with bylaws/rules and regs/policies, and meeting attendance

Step seven: Depending on whether this is an initial application or a reapplication, the MSO may need to gather additional information from primary sources. In general, when physicians apply for medical staff appointment, they must provide the MSO with the names of individuals who can attest to their skill, judgment, and technique.

MSPs and credentials committee members should design and use excellent reference questionnaires to obtain information concerning all medical staff applicants.

Such references are particularly important for specialists with no or little hospital volume. Turn to **Figure 4.1** and **Figure 4.2** on pp. 86 and 87 in Chapter four for more information about professional references.

When an existing medical staff member submits a reappointment application, the MSO must gather information that confirms the practitioner's experience and performance. This information can be collected from internal sources and should include everything the institution knows about the practitioner that could help the credentials committee and MEC determine reappointment eligibility. The MSO also must obtain precise information about the reapplicant's clinical volume at the facility.

Note: Medical staff bylaws and accreditation requirements detail the exact information the MSO must collect from internal and external sources when processing applications.

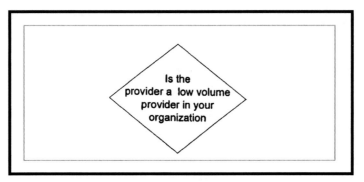

Step eight: After collecting relevant information, the organization must determine whether the applicant or reapplicant is a low- or no-volume provider. A practitioner could fall into one of the following broad low- and no-volume provider categories:

1. The practitioner has no or low volume at your facility and no volume at another inpatient facility. A practitioner who is slowing down his or her practice and no longer engages in clinical activity would fall into this category.

2. The practitioner has no- or low-volume at your facility but engages in significant clinical work in an ambulatory setting or in another healthcare facility. Under these circumstances, the organization must obtain information directly from those facilities to proceed with the appraisal or reappraisal process. Turn to Chapter three for tips on collecting that information.

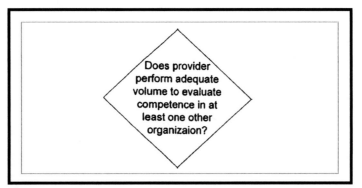

Step nine: If the provider performs satisfactory clinical work at another organization, the MSO should collect volume and performance data from that facility (go to Chapter four for tips about obtaining this important data). Once this information is gathered, the MSO can continue on to step 10 of the appraisal/reappraisal process.

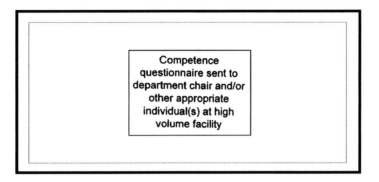

Remember, the burden is always on the practitioner to provide information that is not forthcoming from acceptable alternative sources. See Chapter three for additional information about the physician's obligation to provide your organization with this data.

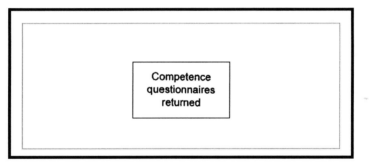

When the MSO receives the required volume and performance information from appropriate sources, the MSP can continue to step 10 of the appraisal/reappraisal process.

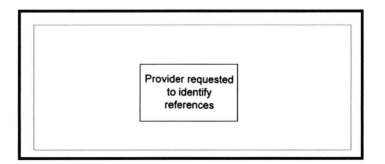

If the MSO determines that the provider does not engage in clinical work at another accredited facility, it must ask the applicant to identify appropriate individuals who can and will provide information concerning his or her current clinical competence.

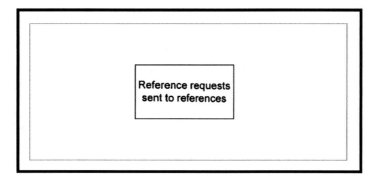

Reference questionnaires should then be sent to those individuals, with a cover letter establishing the importance of a timely and candid response. Turn to **Figure 2.6** on p. 50 for a sample policy on clinical references.

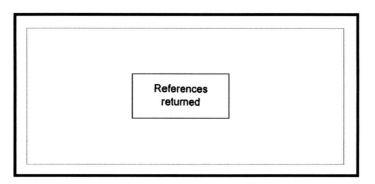

If the references are not returned in a timely manner, the MSO should notify the applicant or reapplicant of the responsibility to obtain required information. A form letter may be useful in this process. See **Figure 3.2** on p. 67 in Chapter three for guidance.

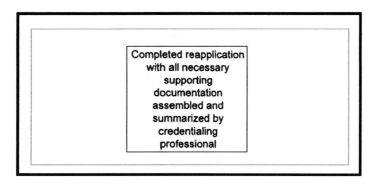

Step 10: Once the MSO collects all of the information it needs to evaluate the application or reapplication, the MSP should summarize that information to present it to the department chair. Turn to **Figure 2.7** on p. 52 for a sample reappointment activity summary.

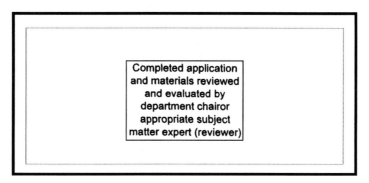

Step 11: The department chair must review the completed application. To carry out this step of the process effectively, the department chair must be trained in the mechanics and substance of application review and evaluation.

The department chair should quickly and thoroughly review the application so as not to unnecessarily prolong or delay the entire appraisal/reappraisal process. Department chairs who fail to review the application in a timely manner risk losing the opportunity to comment on the application prior to its receipt by the medical executive committee (MEC). In most hospitals, the department chair is an MEC member and may be asked to provide his or her commentary at the MEC meeting.

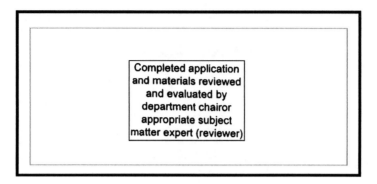

Step 12: Many hospitals now use an expedited or streamlined application and reap-plication review process.

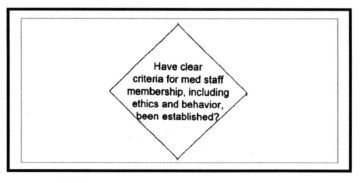

If the department chair and the MSP determine that an application warrants the expedited process, that process begins after the department chair evaluates the application. Turn to **Figure 2.8** on p. 54 for a sample fast-track credentialing policy. This policy can be modified for use within your facility, with the approval of the med-ical staff and board.

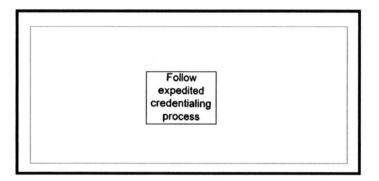

Step 13: Determine whether the medical staff bylaws or associated credentials policies contain objective criteria for medical staff membership, category, and department assignment. These criteria should address clinical volume for category assignment and medical staff membership.

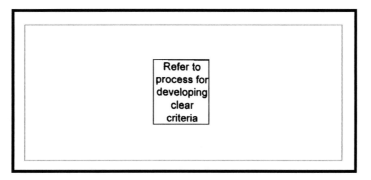

If the organization has not established clear criteria for medical staff membership or has failed to review criteria recently, the issue should be referred to the MEC for consideration and criteria development or revision.

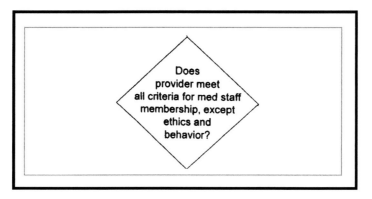

Step 14: If the medical staff bylaws or associated policies contained appropriate criteria for medical staff membership, and for category and departmental assignment, the organization must determine whether the applicant meets the criteria.

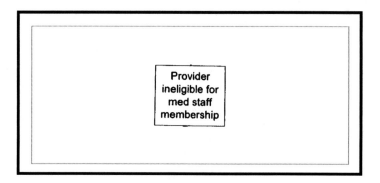

If applicants do not meet the criteria, the MSO should notify them that they are ineligible for medical staff membership or ineligible for assignment to the category of their choice. The department chair or MSP must then decide whether the medical staff bylaws require the hospital to notify the applicants of their right to request a hearing.

Ideally, an applicant or reapplicant who fails to meet the objective criteria for medical staff membership or category assignment would be ineligible to request a hearing because no decision has been made concerning his or her professional performance. The applicant should simply be notified that he or she is ineligible for appointment to the staff or for desired category assignment.

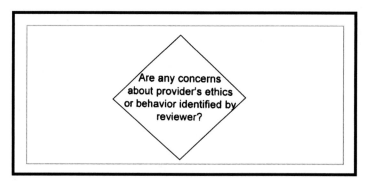

Step 15: The organization must determine whether there are any concerns about the provider's ethics or professional behavior. If such concerns are identified, the MSO or credentials committee must collect information to validate or resolve these concerns.

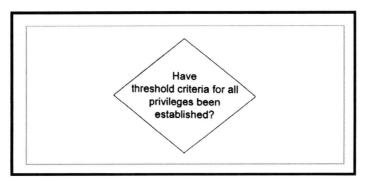

Step 16: The department chair should determine whether the medical staff previously established criteria for the granting of clinical privileges.

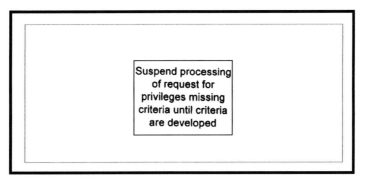

If such criteria have not been established, the department chair should consider whether to continue the appraisal or reappraisal process. If the organization has failed to develop criteria for the requested clinical privileges, the department chair should suspend processing while the relevant medical staff committees develop threshold criteria under which this particular request may be reviewed.

All grants of clinical privilege should consider whether the physician meets certain pre-defined criteria concerning education, training, and experience.

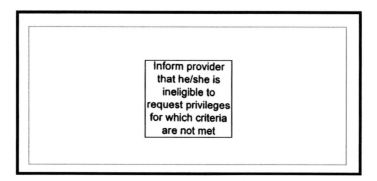

Step 17: If the applicant does not meet the criteria for clinical privileges, the organization must explain that the application will not be considered until it receives evidence demonstrating that the provider meets the criteria. The physician may choose to provide the organization with additional information that demonstrates that he or she does indeed meet the objective criteria concerning education, training, and experience. The physician may also allow his or her request for clinical privileges to expire.

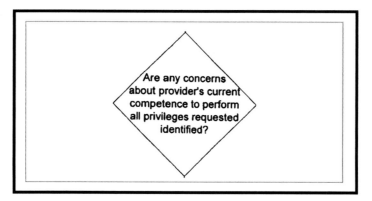

Step 18: The department chair must determine whether the provider is currently clinically competent to perform all requested privileges. To do so, the department chair must evaluate the applicant's skill, judgment, overall professional performance, and results of performance improvement activities. The department chairs should document the evaluation.

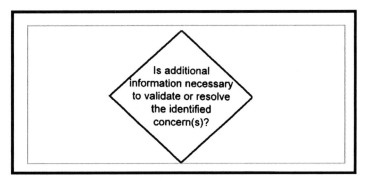

Step 19: If additional information is necessary to validate or resolve concerns about the applicant's competence, the MSO and an appropriate medical staff member (often the chair of the credentials committee or the vice president for medical affairs) should determine what information is needed to validate or resolve the concern.

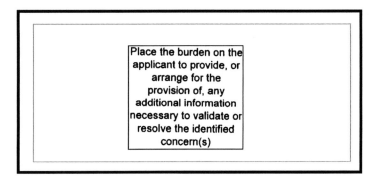

The department chair should place the burden squarely on the applicant to provide or arrange for the provision of additional information to validate or resolve the identified concerns. As indicated previously, when placing the burden on the practitioner, the MSO should send the applicant a letter that specifies the material he or she must submit to the MSO.

If the MSO does not receive the information within the timeframe specified in this letter, it should send the applicant another letter stating that it has terminated the application or reapplication process due to the physician's failure to provide necessary information.

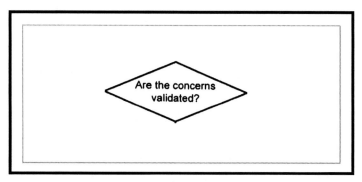

Once the MSO receives the information from the applicant, the organization should review the information to determine whether the previously identified concerns are valid.

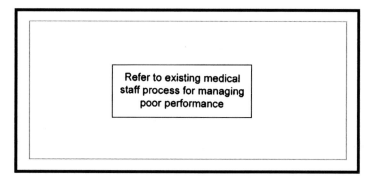

If such concerns are valid, the issue should be referred to the MEC or other process designed to assist in managing poor physician performance. Proceed to the next step of the process if the concerns are not validated and the new information demonstrates that the applicant is indeed currently clinically qualified.

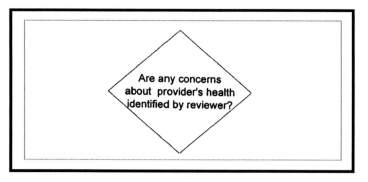

Step 20: The department chair must now consider the applicant's or reapplicant's health status.

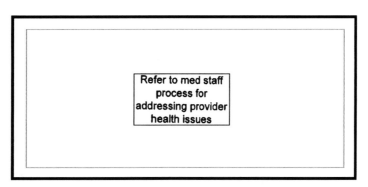

If problems with the provider's health are detected, the department chair should refer the applicant to the medical staff's process for identifying provider health issues—either a physician aide or an impaired physician committee. It is not the department chair's responsibility to conduct an investigation to resolve concerns about a practitioner's health status.

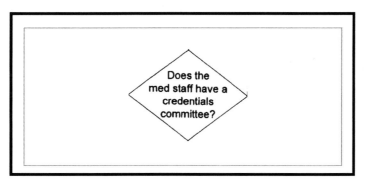

Step 21: If the department chair does not have any concerns about the physician applicant's health status and he or she can attest to the physician's ability to provide health services safely and effectively, the issue should be referred to the credentials committee if such a committee exists.

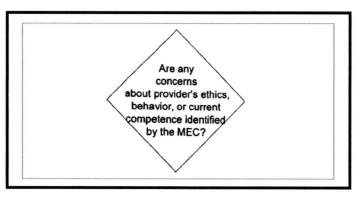

The credentials committee must review the application and identify any concerns about the physician's ethics, behavior, and competence. If the committee identifies such concerns, it should follow the advice discussed in step 19.

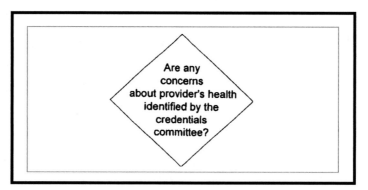

The credentials committee must also determine whether the information on the practitioner's application indicates health problems that could affect his or her ability to deliver quality patient care.

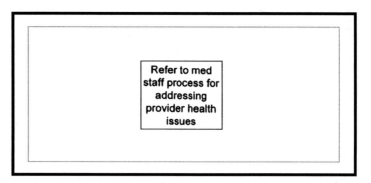

If the credentials committee identifies such concerns, it should refer the application to the process designed by the medical staff to evaluate health issues.

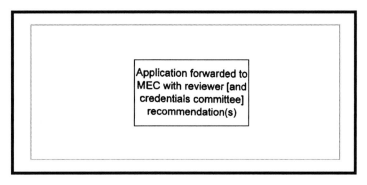

The physician's application should be referred to the MEC in the event that the credentials committee does not have any concerns about his or her ethics, behavior, competence, or health status.

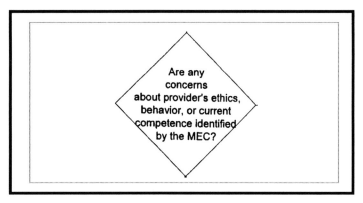

Step 22: If the MEC identifies concerns about the physician applicant's ethics, behavior, competence, or health status, the committee should follow the steps outlined above.

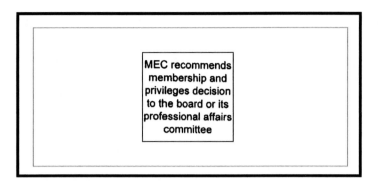

If the MEC does not identify problems with the application, it should submit to the board its recommendation regarding the practitioner's appointment or reappointment to the medical staff, departmental and category assignment, and clinical privileges. The MEC may also submit this recommendation to an authorized subcommittee, which is often referred to as the professional affairs committee.

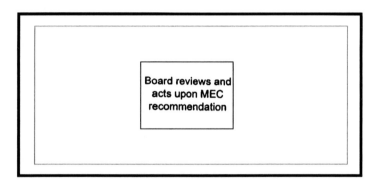

Step 23: The board, or its appropriate subcommittee, would then act on the MEC's recommendation.

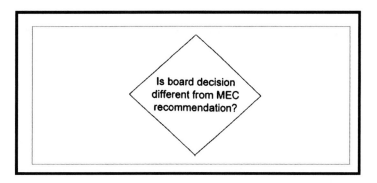

Step 24: If the board's decision varies from that of the MEC, the issue should be referred to a joint conference between board officers and medical staff officers for further consideration.

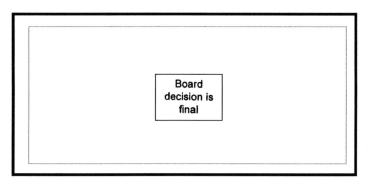

Step 25: If the board's decision is in accordance with the MEC's recommendation, the decision is final (provided that the applicant does not request a fair hearing if the recommendation and final decision are adverse).

FIGURE 2.1

APPLICATION FOR MEDICAL STAFF APPOINTMENT AND CLINICAL PRIVILEGES

Note: Please print or use typewriter. All professional information (including addresses) must be included for application to be considered complete. All time periods must be accounted for. Do not leave any item blank. Please write "not applicable" or "NA" where necessary.

NAME: _____
       LAST   FIRST   MI   SUFFIX   TITLE

OTHER NAME(S) USED: _____
       LAST   FIRST   MI   SUFFIX   TITLE

GROUP NAME: _____

PRIMARY OFFICE ADDRESS: _____
       STREET   CITY/STATE   ZIP   PHONE   FAX

SECOND OFFICE: _____
       STREET   CITY/STATE   ZIP   PHONE   FAX

HOME ADDRESS: _____
       STREET   CITY/STATE   ZIP   PHONE

ANSWERING SERVICE: _____
                              (if applicable)

DATE OF BIRTH: _____ PLACE OF BIRTH: _____ UPIN #: _____ MEDICAID# _____

CITIZENSHIP: _____ ALIEN STATUS: _____ ADMISSION #: _____

WORK AUTH. EXP.: _____ SOCIAL SECURITY #: _____

FOREIGN LANGUAGES:

LANGUAGE	SPEAK	READ	WRITE

AMERICAN SIGN LANGUAGE: ❑ Yes ❑ No

| FIGURE 2.1 | APPLICATION FOR MEDICAL STAFF APPOINTMENT AND CLINICAL PRIVILEGES (CONT.) |

I AM APPLYING FOR MEMBERSHIP ON THE MEDICAL STAFF IN THE STAFF CATEGORY OF:
❑ Active   ❑ Associate   ❑ Consulting   ❑ Courtesy   ❑ Emeritus

AND REQUEST PRIVILEGES IN THE DEPARTMENT(S) OF:
❑ Anesthesia   ❑ Emergency Services   ❑ Family Practice   ❑ Medicine   ❑ Obstetrics/Gynecology
❑ Ophthalmology   ❑ Otolaryngology   ❑ Pathology   ❑ Psychiatry   ❑ Radiology   ❑ Surgery

SUBSPECIALTY: _____

EDUCATION:
TYPE: (U) UNDERGRADUATE   (P) PROFESSIONAL   (O) OTHER

TYPE	INSTITUTION AND ADDRESS	DEGREE	DATES (TO/FROM)
			/
			/
			/
			/
			/
			/

GRADUATE MEDICAL TRAINING:
TYPE: (I) INTERNSHIP   (R) RESIDENCY   (F) FELLOWSHIP   (O) OTHER CLINICAL:

TYPE	INSTITUTION AND ADDRESS	PROGRAM DIRECTOR	DEGREE	DATES (TO/FROM)
				/
				/
				/
				/
				/
				/
				/

Were all graduate medical training programs successfully completed?   ❑ Yes   ❑ No
If no, provide explanation on separate sheet.
Chief residency dates: (From/To) _____

| FIGURE 2.1 | APPLICATION FOR MEDICAL STAFF APPOINTMENT AND CLINICAL PRIVILEGES (CONT.) |

PROFESSIONAL REFERENCES

List at least two medical or health care professionals and as many more as you like, not including relatives, current partners, or associates in practice. Provide current complete addresses. References will be evaluated according to the extent of their direct clinical observation of your work and other knowledge of you.

NAME	ADDRESS	RELATIONSHIP

PROFESSIONAL LICENSURE (Include all past and present, including current, lapsed, suspended, revoked, restricted, voluntary, or involuntary. Specify type, i.e., MD, DDS, DO, DPM. Attach copies.)

STATE LICENSE	DATE ISSUE	LICENSE NUMBER	TYPE	EXPIRATION DATE

ECFMG (if applicable)

NUMBER	DATE ISSUED	EXPIRATION DATE

CONTROLLED SUBSTANCE REGISTRATION

TYPE: (S) STATE (F) FEDERAL

STATE/AGENCY	DATE ISSUE	NUMBER	TYPE	EXPIRATION DATE

| FIGURE 2.1 | APPLICATION FOR *MEDICAL STAFF APPOINTMENT AND CLINICAL PRIVILEGES (CONT.)* |

SPECIALTY BOARD CERTIFICATION

1. Are you currently board certified in any specialty/subspecialty? ❏ Yes   ❏ No
2. Have you ever been examined by a specialty board, but
   failed to pass the examination? ❏ Yes   ❏ No

If not board certified, indicate any of the following that apply: _____
❏ I have taken examination, results pending for _____ board
❏ I have taken Part I and am eligible for Part II of the _____ exam
❏ I intend to sit for the boards on _____ date
❏ I do not plan to take boards

FIELD CERTIFIED IN	CERTIFYING BOARD NAME	DATE CERT.	DATE RECEIVED CERT.	EXPIRATION DATE	CAN TAKE EXAM UNTIL

OTHER CERTIFICATIONS: (Basic life support and/or other clinical certifications)

TYPE	SPONSOR	DATE CERT.	EXPIRATION DATE

Do you hold CPR instructor certification? ❏ Yes   ❏ No

APPLICATION FOR MEDICAL STAFF APPOINTMENT AND CLINICAL PRIVILEGES (CONT.)

HOSPITAL STAFF APPOINTMENTS (List in chronological order since completion of postgraduate education. Include all organizations (past and present) of which you are or were an employee, associate, practitioner, or member of the medical staff for purposes of providing patient care.

HOSPITAL & ADDRESS	DEPARTMENT/CHIEF	STAFF STATUS	DATES (FROM/TO)
			/
			/
			/
			/
			/
			/
			/

ADMINISTRATIVE POSITIONS (Include all past and present) List all administrative positions held on other hospital staffs and with other medical affiliations, corporations, military assignments, or government agencies. Attach a separate sheet if more space is needed.

INSTITUTION & ADDRESS	POSITION	RESPONSIBILITIES	DATES (FROM/TO)
			/
			/
			/
			/
			/
			/
			/

APPLICATION FOR MEDICAL STAFF APPOINTMENT AND CLINICAL PRIVILEGES (CONT.)

PRACTICE HISTORY Include all professional affiliations, including private practice and current status.

TYPE: (S) Solo   (P) Partnership   (G) Single specialty group
(MS) Multispecialty Group   (HMO) HMO Employment

TYPE	PRACTICE NAME & ADDRESS	SUPERVISOR	DATES (FROM/TO)
			/
			/
			/
			/
			/
			/
			/

Do you have any material interest either directly or through family or business partners in any nursing homes, laboratories, pharmacies, medical equipment or supply houses or other businesses to which patients from this hospital might be referred or recommended?   ❑ Yes   ❑ No

MANAGED CARE AFFILIATIONS (past & present) List all managed care affiliations held.

ORGANIZATION & ADDRESS	SPECIALTY	DATES (FROM/TO)
		/
		/
		/
		/

ACADEMIC APPOINTMENTS (past & present)

INSTITUTION & ADDRESS	DEPARTMENT	RANK	DATES (FROM/TO)
			/
			/
			/
			/

FIGURE 2.1

APPLICATION FOR MEDICAL STAFF APPOINTMENT AND CLINICAL PRIVILEGES (CONT.)

PROFESSIONAL LIABILITY INSURANCE

Include name of all carriers for last ten years, including address, city, state and zip code, policy number, and amount of coverage.

CARRIER/ADDRESS	POLICY #	AMOUNT	DATES OF COVERAGE

Have there ever been or are there currently pending any claims, settlements or judgments against you?   ❏ Yes   ❏ No

Has your professional liability insurance carrier(s) excluded any specific area of practice, or terminated or denied coverage?   ❏ Yes   ❏ No

If the answer to any of the above questions is yes, please provide a full explanation of the details of each matter on a separate sheet and attach. The explanation must include the name of the court in which the suit was filed, the caption and docket number of the case, the name and address of your attorney, and all other relevant details. Include suits in which a judgment or settlement was made against a professional corporation of which you are/were a member, shareholder, or employee in any matter in which you were involved in the patient's care.

CLINICAL PERFORMANCE

If the answer is YES to the following question, on a separate attached sheet please provide full details including names and addresses of physicians/hospitals involved.

Do you have any condition which could compromise your ability to perform any of the mental and physical functions related to the specific clinical privileges you are requesting and the duties and responsibilities of appointment including emergency coverage?   ❏ Yes   ❏ No

If yes, please provide full details on a separate sheet, including a description of any accommodations that could reasonably be made to facilitate your performance of such functions without risk of compromise. Regardless of how this question is answered, the application will be processed in the usual manner. If you have answered this question affirmatively, and are found to be professionally qualified for medical staff appointment and the clinical privileges requested, you will be given an opportunity to meet with the physician's health task force to determine what accommodations are necessary or feasible to allow you to practice safely.

FIGURE 2.1

APPLICATION FOR MEDICAL STAFF APPOINTMENT AND CLINICAL PRIVILEGES (CONT.)

DISCIPLINARY ACTIONS

Have any of the following ever been, or are any currently in the process of being, investigated, challenged, denied, revoked, terminated, suspended, reduced, limited, relinquished, placed on probation or not renewed, voluntarily or involuntarily? If yes, please provide full explanation below or on a separate sheet.

Medical license ❑ Yes ❑ No

Other health related professional registration/license
(e.g., federal or state controlled substance permit) ❑ Yes ❑ No

Academic appointment ❑ Yes ❑ No

Membership on any hospital medical staff ❑ Yes ❑ No

Clinical privileges at any hospital ❑ Yes ❑ No

Prerogatives/rights on any medical staff ❑ Yes ❑ No

Other institutional affiliation, status, or privileges ❑ Yes ❑ No

Health-related professional society membership or
fellowship/board certification or ECFMG Certification ❑ Yes ❑ No

Have you ever been convicted of or pleaded guilty or
no contest to any criminal charges (other than motor
vehicle speeding violations)? ❑ Yes ❑ No

Have you ever been convicted of or pleaded no contest
to a drug or alcohol related offense? ❑ Yes ❑ No

Have you ever been suspended, sanctioned or otherwise
restricted from participating in any private, federal or
state health insurance program (e.g., Medicare or Medicaid),
or by a PSRO, PRO, or similar federal or state health agency? ❑ Yes ❑ No

Have you ever voluntarily relinquished, withdrawn, or failed
to proceed with an application for any of the above in order
to avoid an adverse action or to preclude an investigation
or while under investigation relating to professional conduct? ❑ Yes ❑ No

FIGURE 2.2

THE NEW CREDENTIALING STANDARD: TEN STEPS TO CREDENTIALING EXCELLENCE

① **Standard one: Lifetime licensure history**

Summary: Verify each physician's or medical staff applicant's lifetime licensure history. Check all licenses currently held by the applicant across all healthcare disciplines (including allied disciplines) and previous licenses no longer held by the applicant.

Rationale: A growing number of applicants may have had one ore more of their state-issued licenses revoked, suspended, or otherwise restricted. For example, some medical staff candidates possess a valid license to practice medicine, osteopathy, oral surgery, or podiatry but may have had a license to practice as a pharmacists or registered nurse revoked or restricted.

How to comply: First, ask the applicant a series of questions about his or her lifetime licensure history. Second, verify the applicant's answers, history, and any other relevant information collected.

② **Standard two: Lifetime medical education and training history**

Summary: Verify the applicant's lifetime medical education and training history, including all medical, osteopathic, podiatric, dental, or other schools attended, as well as all approved or unapproved residency and fellowship programs.

Rationale: A growing number of applicants are unable to complete medical school during the routine four years. Thus, they find it necessary to enroll in more than one medical school prior to obtaining their medical degree or enroll in more than one residency, fellowship, or other training program—whether such training has been approved by a U.S.-accredited body or not. Credentials committees should have access to this information.

Similarly, some physicians begin their medical education at an offshore medical school that is not approved by an accrediting organization in the United States. These medical schools may have more lenient entrance and graduation requirements than the minimal standards required by accredited U.S. medical schools.

In addition, many physicians find it necessary to transfer from one residency program to another. While most do so at their option, a small number of physicians change residency programs when they are not offered a contract for post-graduate years two, three, or four.

How to comply: First, ask the applicant a series of questions about his or her medical school education, residencies, fellowships and other training. Second, verify the applicant's answers, history, and any other relevant information collected.

③ **Standard three: Malpractice insurance and 10 year history**

Summary: Check the applicant's current malpractice policy and previous 10 year malpractice history, including claims, lawsuits, and settlements. (Include those brought against the physician's professional corporation or incorporated practice.)

Rationale: Although the presence or absence of a malpractice suit indicates little about a practitioner's current clinical competence, malpractice suits may indicate potential problems if such suits occur in large numbers, are clustered within a certain diagnosis or procedure, or result in extremely high court awards.

THE NEW CREDENTIALING STANDARD:
TEN STEPS TO CREDENTIALING EXCELLENCE (CONT.)

FIGURE 2.2

How to comply: First, ask the application a series of questions about his or her malpractice history. Second, request a copy of the current policy fact sheet on the application. Then verify the applicant's answers, history, and any other relevant information collected.

(4) Standard four: Specialty board status

Summary: Verify the applicant's specialty board status. Obtain information on admissibility to take the exam, components of the exam currently taken, sections passed or failed, as well as the number of times the applicant took the exam. Confirm either no status or certification.

Rationale: While the applicant's certification or lack of certification does not, in and of itself, indicate clinical competence, certification does show that the applicant has demonstrated a complete grasp of the knowledge and skills necessary to perform effectively.

One excellent benchmark of a physician's medical knowledge and skills is whether he or she took an exam or received certification from a recognized specialty board. This benchmark should be evaluated by all individuals undertaking credentialing.

For an applicant who did not pass part one or part two of the examination over a prolonged period, the credentials committee should carefully evaluate the applicant based on references received from a significant number of individuals with direct knowledge of the applicant's current clinical abilities.

How to comply: First, ask the applicant a series of detailed questions about his or her specialty board status. Second, verify the applicant's answers, history, and any other relevant information collected.

(5) Standard five: Sanctions and disciplinary actions

Summary: Investigate all sanctions or disciplinary actions taken, recommended, or pending against an applicant by a hospital, health system, components of a health system, freestanding ambulatory care facility, any branch of the federal or state government, specialty board, or managed care organization.

Rationale: Currently, institutions—such as the Department of Justice, Office of Inspector General, Drug Enforcement Agency (DEA), state-specific Controlled Dangerous Substance agencies, and Food and Drug Administration—have taken approximately 38,600 disciplinary actions against more than 20,000 physicians. In addition, thousands of physicians have been disciplined by private organizations, such as hospitals, managed care organizations, surgicenters, ambulatory care centers, and specialty boards.

While more than 90 percent of the physicians in the U.S. have never had any disciplinary action taken against them, according to the Public Citizen's Health Research Group, healthcare managers have more reason today than ever to be concerned about identifying physicians with problem backgrounds. A history of committing fraud or jeopardizing patient safety is not only dangerous to patients, but fraught with legal liability risks as well. Physician incompetence can cost hospitals thousands or millions of dollars in federal and state fines, lawsuits, and restitution. At worst, an incompetent physician or staff member may cause a patient death.

How to comply: First, ask the applicant a series of questions about his or her history of sanctions or disciplinary actions. Second, require a copy of his or her DEA certificate. Then verify the applicant's answers, history, and any other relevant information collected.

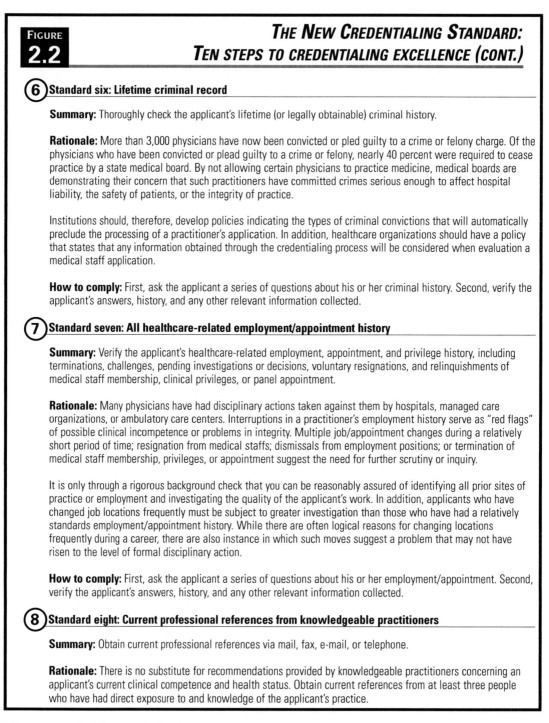

FIGURE
2.2

THE NEW CREDENTIALING STANDARD:
TEN STEPS TO CREDENTIALING EXCELLENCE (CONT.)

⑥ Standard six: Lifetime criminal record

Summary: Thoroughly check the applicant's lifetime (or legally obtainable) criminal history.

Rationale: More than 3,000 physicians have now been convicted or pled guilty to a crime or felony charge. Of the physicians who have been convicted or plead guilty to a crime or felony, nearly 40 percent were required to cease practice by a state medical board. By not allowing certain physicians to practice medicine, medical boards are demonstrating their concern that such practitioners have committed crimes serious enough to affect hospital liability, the safety of patients, or the integrity of practice.

Institutions should, therefore, develop policies indicating the types of criminal convictions that will automatically preclude the processing of a practitioner's application. In addition, healthcare organizations should have a policy that states that any information obtained through the credentialing process will be considered when evaluation a medical staff application.

How to comply: First, ask the applicant a series of questions about his or her criminal history. Second, verify the applicant's answers, history, and any other relevant information collected.

⑦ Standard seven: All healthcare-related employment/appointment history

Summary: Verify the applicant's healthcare-related employment, appointment, and privilege history, including terminations, challenges, pending investigations or decisions, voluntary resignations, and relinquishments of medical staff membership, clinical privileges, or panel appointment.

Rationale: Many physicians have had disciplinary actions taken against them by hospitals, managed care organizations, or ambulatory care centers. Interruptions in a practitioner's employment history serve as "red flags" of possible clinical incompetence or problems in integrity. Multiple job/appointment changes during a relatively short period of time; resignation from medical staffs; dismissals from employment positions; or termination of medical staff membership, privileges, or appointment suggest the need for further scrutiny or inquiry.

It is only through a rigorous background check that you can be reasonably assured of identifying all prior sites of practice or employment and investigating the quality of the applicant's work. In addition, applicants who have changed job locations frequently must be subject to greater investigation than those who have had a relatively standards employment/appointment history. While there are often logical reasons for changing locations frequently during a career, there are also instance in which such moves suggest a problem that may not have risen to the level of formal disciplinary action.

How to comply: First, ask the applicant a series of questions about his or her employment/appointment. Second, verify the applicant's answers, history, and any other relevant information collected.

⑧ Standard eight: Current professional references from knowledgeable practitioners

Summary: Obtain current professional references via mail, fax, e-mail, or telephone.

Rationale: There is no substitute for recommendations provided by knowledgeable practitioners concerning an applicant's current clinical competence and health status. Obtain current references from at least three people who have had direct exposure to and knowledge of the applicant's practice.

THE NEW CREDENTIALING STANDARD:
TEN STEPS TO CREDENTIALING EXCELLENCE (CONT.)

References should not be provided solely by the applicant. We recommend obtaining references from individuals within the practitioner's specialty, as well as people who have worked in related specialties. One reference should be an individual who can verify the approximate number, type, and location of patients; and procedures performed and diagnoses treated. Some examples of references are: director of the applicant's residency and/or fellowship program, chair of the clinical department at the facility where the individual most recently practiced.

If the applicant is applying for a position in which significant nursing or allied health interaction is required, get references from managers who can provide information about the practitioner's overall performance and ability to relate to others on the healthcare team.

How to comply: First, ask the applicant a series of questions about his or her professional references. Second, verify the applicant's answers, history, and any other relevant information collected. Seek out current professional references who are familiar with the applicant and his or her work.

⑨ Standard nine: Clinical activity for the past six to 12 months

Summary: Require a summary report of the applicant's past six to 12 months of clinical activity (including the approximate number, type, and location of patients treated) as part of the medical staff application. For applicants who have had little clinical activity, obtain the full 12-month report.

Rationale: While references attesting to excellent current clinical competence are one of the most important components of the credentialing process, references alone do not provide a complete picture of the applicant's competency. It is necessary to link professional references to a report demonstrating the applicant's actual clinical work. References attesting to excellent judgment in the area of surgery—coupled with a report demonstrating that the applicant has performed the type of surgery in question and an adequate number of surgeries—permit a credentialing committee to formulate a complete recommendation.

Conversely, if an applicant displays significant experience in a particular field but does not back the experience with professional references, that applicant has failed to demonstrate current clinical competence.

You may give the applicant's references a precise list of the clinical activities that the practitioner may possibly perform at your facility. Then ask the references to evaluate the applicant's judgment, skill, technique, and professional performance in those areas of clinical privilege. Nothing, however, completely substitutes a report outlining the general scope of the applicant's clinical experience during the preceding six to 12 months.

How to comply: First, ask the applicant a series of questions about his or her clinical activity. Request a summary of the physician's clinical activity covering the past six to 12 months. Then verify the applicant's answers, history, and any other relevant information collected.

⑩ Standard 10: Comparison of applicant-provided information and verified information

Summary: Summarize and compare all the applicant's collected and verified information for review by physician leaders, committees, and the board.

Rationale: The task of reviewing and cross-checking information in the applicant's file is complex and time-consuming. Therefore, a clear report of the information is necessary. A committee will rarely have time to

---

FIGURE
2.2

THE NEW CREDENTIALING STANDARD:
TEN STEPS TO CREDENTIALING EXCELLENCE (CONT.)

carefully review and cross-reference an average credentials file against such documents as the American Medical Association Profile to search for previous state licenses or ones not listed by the applicant. Nor will committee members have time to check both the National Practitioner Data Bank (NPDB) report and the Fraud and Abuse Control Information System report to determine if any of the candidate's licenses were ever subject to disciplinary action.

How to comply: The committee should assign the task of summary and preliminary evaluation of the applicant's credentials to a person with excellent analytical skills, an eye for detail, and a nose for discrepancies. This person might be an experienced medical services professional, vice president of medical affairs, or a conscientious committee chair. This person should probably not be a department chair, credentials committee member, medical executive committee member, or board member.

The job of summarizing and comparing the collected information requires patience and skill. An administrative review should be made, beginning with a brief narrative that describes the applicant, his or her education, training, previous experience, and areas of practice. The summary should also identify any red flags, discrepancies, or unusual aspects to the applicant's history.

The administrative review should also include the following:

1. Certification status
2. Licensure status
3. DEA status
4. Malpractice insurance and experience
5. Disciplinary actions on record
6. Information from the NPDB
7. American Medical Association Profile or equivalent information
8. Criminal background check issues (if any)
9. Prior hospitals or healthcare organizations
10. A brief summary of references (including the names of individual references)

Any problems associated with collecting information for the file should be discussed with committee members.

FIGURE 2.3

INSTRUCTIONS FOR COMPLETING AN APPLICATION FOR MEDICAL STAFF APPOINTMENT

APPLICANT REQUIREMENTS

The applicant
- must return the completed medical staff appointment application to the medical staff office within 30 days of receipt
- must print or type all information included on the completed application
- complete all spaces on the application; if an area is not applicable, the applicant must write, "N/A"
- must provide all addresses and phone numbers requested
- include month and year for all dates requested
- sign the completed application and accompanying statements

Please include the application fee and copies of the following documents when returning your completed application:
- Your current [State] license
- Your current [State] controlled substance registration
- Your current federal DEA controlled substance registration
- Current professional liability certificate of insurance
- Certificates transcribed into English if any professional education training was obtained outside of the U.S.

Please personally present either of the following (original) documents to the medical staff office:
- U.S. passport, certificate of U.S. citizenship, certificate of naturalization, current foreign passport with attached employment authorization, or alien registration card with photograph,
- State-issued drivers license or U.S. military card AND social security card, certified birth certificate, or current INS employment authorization

APPLICATION INSTRUCTIONS

Page 1—General information

Every applicant must furnish the following complete information:
- **Personal information**—local home and office addresses and telephone numbers, date of birth, foreign language facility, citizenship, and visa status.
- Please check the box that corresponds to the department(s) and subspecialty(s) for which you are requesting privileges.

Page 2—Membership, privileges, education and training, and references

Every applicant must furnish the following complete information:
- **Membership, department, and affiliation status**—department affiliation, staff category assignment, and specific requested clinical privileges.
- **Educational background, training, and experience**—undergraduate, professional school, and postgraduate training, including the name of each institution attended, degrees granted, programs

---

FIGURE 2.3

INSTRUCTIONS FOR COMPLETING AN APPLICATION FOR MEDICAL STAFF APPOINTMENT (CONT.)

completed, dates attended, and, for post-graduate training, names of practitioners responsible for monitoring the applicant's performance.

- **Professional references**—the application must include the names of at least three (3) professional references who are not newly associated, planning to partner with the applicant in professional practice, or personally related to him; who have personal knowledge of the applicant's current clinical ability, ethical character, health status, and ability to work cooperatively with others; and who will provide specific written comments on these matters at the hospital's request.

The named individuals must have acquired the requisite knowledge through recent (within the past three years) observation of the applicant's professional performance over a period of time. At least one reference should come from a colleague in the applicant's specialty.

Pages 4, 5, and 6—Licensure, registration, certification, and appointment

Every applicant must furnish the following complete information:

- **Licensure and registration**—all past and currently valid medical, dental, podiatric, and other professional licenses, permits, and certifications; and federal and state controlled substance registration, including issue and expiration date. A copy of the current federal registration must accompany the application.
- **Specialty certification/recertification**—specialty or subspecialty board certification, recertification, or status in the certification process according to the particular board's requirements.

Pages 7, 8, and 9—Practice history, managed care affiliations, academic appointments, liability insurance, and clinical performance

Every applicant must furnish the following complete information:

- **Affiliations**—office locations; names and addresses of other practitioners with whom the applicant is or was associated, including dates of that association; names and locations of all other hospitals, clinics, or healthcare organizations where or through which the applicant provides or provided clinical services, including dates of each affiliation, status held, and general scope of clinical privileges. Please include information regarding affiliations with managed care organizations.
- **Academic appointments**—past and present academic appointments, including name and address of the institution, department, rank, and dates of the appointment.
- **Professional liability insurance coverage**—past and current professional liability insurance coverage, and malpractice claims history and experience (claims, suits and settlements made, concluded, and pending), including the names and addresses of present and past insurance carriers.
- **Health status***—any previous or current mental/physical problem or disability (including alcohol or drug dependency) that affects the ability to provide safe patient care or that may be expected to progress within the next two years to the point of affecting the applicant's ability in terms of skill, attitude, or judgment; hospitalizations for any mental/physical problem or disability during the past five (5) years.
- **Actions**—all pending or completed actions involving denial, revocation, cancellation, suspension, reduction, limitation, or probation of any of the following, and any nonrenewal or relinquishment of or

*All healthcare organizations must comply with the Americans with Disabilities Act.

FIGURE 2.3

INSTRUCTIONS FOR COMPLETING AN APPLICATION FOR MEDICAL STAFF APPOINTMENT (CONT.)

withdrawal of an application for any of the following to avoid investigation or possible disciplinary or adverse action:

— license or certificate to practice any health-related profession in any state or country

— federal- or state-controlled substance registration

— membership or fellowship in local, state, or national health or scientific professional organizations

— faculty appointment at any medical or other professional school

— appointment or employment status, prerogatives, or clinical privileges at any healthcare facility

— professional liability insurance

— any current criminal charges (other than motor vehicle violations) and any drug or alcohol-related charges (including motor vehicle violations) pending against the applicant and any past charges, including their resolution

Conditions of application and representation of applicant

By signing the completed application for medical staff membership, the applicant

• attests to the correctness and completeness of all information furnished, and acknowledges that any misstatement, misrepresentation, or omission from the application, whether intentional or not, constitutes grounds for denial of appointment or for summary dismissal from the medical staff in the event that appointment and privileges have been granted prior to the discovery of the misstatement, misrepresentation, or omission

• signifies the applicant's willingness to appear for interview in connection with the application, and willingness to abide by the hospital's medical staff bylaws, medical staff manuals, and hospital policies if granted appointment clinical privileges, and to abide by the terms thereof in all matters relating to consideration of the application without regard to whether appointment privileges are granted

• agrees to maintain an ethical practice and provide continuous care to his or her patients

• agrees to notify, promptly and in writing, the medical staff office of any change made or proposed in the status of his or her professional license or permit to practice; federal- or state-controlled substance registration; professional liability insurance coverage; membership or employment status or clinical privileges at other institutions, facilities, or organizations, and status of current or initiation of new malpractice claims

• authorizes hospital representatives to consult with his or her prior associates, including insurance carriers, who may have information bearing on his or her professional or ethical qualifications and competence, and consents to the hospitals inspecting all documents that may be material to evaluation of said qualifications and competence

• releases from liability all those who—in good faith and without malice—review, act on, or provide information regarding the applicant's background, experience, clinical competence, professional ethics, utilization practice patterns, character, health status, and other qualifications for medical staff appointment and clinical privileges

• sign and date the "acknowledgement of the practitioner" section on the last page of the form

• return this form in its entirety to the medical staff office

Note: *Our [medical staff services director] will review the information submitted on this form and ensure that it is complete. The verification process will begin once the application is deemed complete. You will be notified if more information is required. The completed application, together with the supporting documentation, will be transmitted to the appropriate department chair for review and recommendation.*

FIGURE 2.4

APPLICATION COMPLETION CHECKLIST

Applicant's name: _____ Application #: _____

Item	Yes	No	Comments
Personal information 1. Complete?			
Self-declared specialty 2. Complete?			
3. Does specialty correlate with applicant's training and/or certification?			
Current practice 4. Is practitioner's practice located in the hospital's service area?			
Membership/department affiliation/status 5. Is membership status and department affiliation indicated?			
6. Does this request coincide with the bylaws requirements, that applicant's specialty, department rules and regulations?			
Clinical privileges 7. Complete?			
8. Does the privilege area coincide with the applicant's training and/or certification?			
Licensure/registration 9. Complete?			
10. Copy of current [state] license?			
11. Copy of current [state] controlled substance registration?			
12. Copy of current federal DEA registration?			

| FIGURE 2.4 | APPLICATION COMPLETION CHECKLIST (CONT.) | | |

Item	Yes	No	Comments
Professional liability insurance 13. Copy of current certificate?			
14. Does policy show coverage of at least $1 million/ $3 million (hospital specific)?			
15. Is insurance carrier on the approved list?			
16. Does general coverage include requested clinical privi- leges?			
17. Is there complete information on professional liability carriers from residency to present?			
Certification 18. If certification required, is the practitioner board certi- fied?			
19. If an FMG/IMG, is information on ECGMG certification complete? Has the practitioner included a copy of his or her ECGMG certification?			
Education/training 20. Complete?			
21. Was training sequential from medical school, through internship, residency, and fellowship?			
22. If an FMG/IMG, are there copies of education certificates translated into English?			
Continuing medical education 23. If "special" privileges, is the required documentation of training present?			
Medical practice affiliations 24. Complete?			
25. Are there practice affiliations from residency to present?			

FIGURE 2.4	APPLICATION COMPLETION CHECKLIST (CONT.)

Item	Yes	No	Comments
Hospital affiliations 26. Complete?			
27. Are there hospital affiliations from residency to present?			
Professional references 28. Complete?			
29. Is at least one reference in the applicant's specialty?			
Questions 30. Is an explanation provided wherever indicated?			
31. Is the explanation complete?			
History 32. Can you track the applicant's career from leaving medical school to the present?			
33. Are all periods of time (months/years) accounted for?			
34. Can you identify that the physician practiced in each state in which he or she was licensed?			
Administrative 35. Are all release forms signed and dated?			

❑ **Application complete**   ❑ **Application incomplete**

Complete = all blanks are filled with an answer or N/A, and all information requested on the application is provided, including names, dates, addresses, and phone numbers.

Comments: _____

_____

Signature—Evaluation completed by: _____ Date: _____
       ❑ Agree   ❑ Disagree
Signature—Department chair: _____ Date: _____
Comments: _____

_____

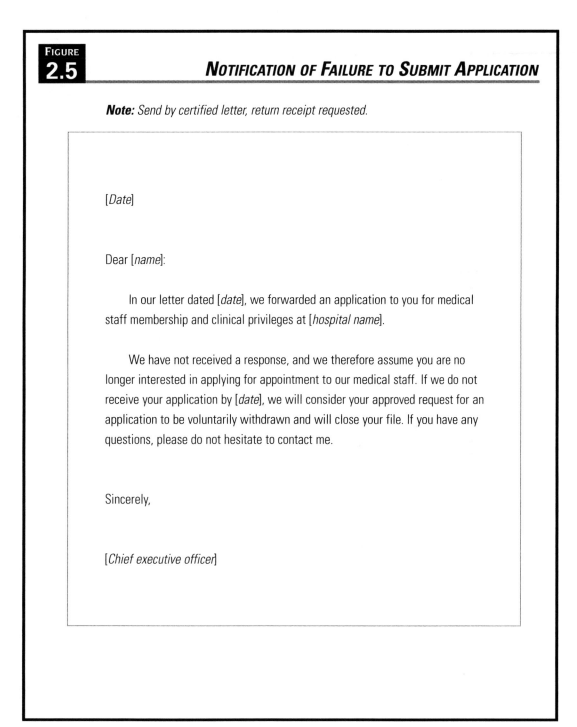

FIGURE 2.5

NOTIFICATION OF FAILURE TO SUBMIT APPLICATION

Note: *Send by certified letter, return receipt requested.*

[*Date*]

Dear [*name*]:

In our letter dated [*date*], we forwarded an application to you for medical staff membership and clinical privileges at [*hospital name*].

We have not received a response, and we therefore assume you are no longer interested in applying for appointment to our medical staff. If we do not receive your application by [*date*], we will consider your approved request for an application to be voluntarily withdrawn and will close your file. If you have any questions, please do not hesitate to contact me.

Sincerely,

[*Chief executive officer*]

| FIGURE 2.6 | POLICY ON CLINICAL REFERENCES |

It is the policy of this institution to process applications for appointment and/or clinical privileges only after receipt of acceptable clinical references (either a completed questionnaire or other) by the institution. Such references must be provided by individuals knowledgeable about the applicant's past clinical and professional activities. The application must include references from the applicant's immediate past or current practice settings (such as residency, current hospital, managed care organization, or immediate past hospital or managed care organization). This institution requires references from at least three of the individuals designated below.

Note: In the event this institution does not receive references from the designated individuals, processing of the application will cease and the medical staff services director and credentials chair will review the application to determine further action.

Specialty	References required
Allergy and immunology	Internist, emergency department physician, and allergist
Anesthesiology	Chief of surgery, operating room supervisor, anesthesiologist
Colon and rectal surgery	Anesthesiologist, operating room supervisor, pathologist, radiologist, colon/rectal surgeon
Dentistry	Pediatrician, family physician, dentist
Dermatology	Internist, family physician, dermatologist
Emergency medicine	Surgeon, internist/cardiologist, emergency department supervisor, emergency medicine physician
Family practice	Emergency department physician, director of nursing, internist, family physician
Internal medicine	Cardiologist, director of nursing, chief of surgery, internist
Neurological surgery	Anesthesiologist, operating room supervisor, emergency department physician, director of nursing, neurosurgeon
Nuclear medicine	Radiologist, pathologist, head technician, nuclear medicine physician
Obstetrics and gynecology	Anesthesiologist, pediatrician, OB/GYN
Ophthalmology	Anesthesiologist, family physician, operating room supervisor, ophthalmologist
Oral and maxillofacial surgery	Anesthesiologist, chief of surgery, oral and maxillofacial surgeon

FIGURE
2.6

POLICY ON CLINICAL REFERENCES (CONT.)

Specialty	References required
Orthopedic surgery	Anesthesiologist, operating room supervisor, radiologist, orthopedist
Otolaryngology	Anesthesiologist, operating room supervisor, family physician, otolaryngologist
Pathology	Surgery, internist, director of pathology
Pediatrics	Pediatric unit director, internist, emergency department physician, pediatrician
Plastic surgery	Anesthesiologist, operating room supervisor, emergency department physician, plastic surgeon
Psychology	Internist, family physician, director of nursing, psychologist
Psychiatry and neurology	Internist, emergency department physician, nursing supervisor, neurologist
Radiology	Orthopedic surgeon, emergency department physician, internist, radiologist
Surgery	Orthopedic surgeon, emergency department physician, internist, general surgeon
Thoracic surgery	Orthopedic surgeon, emergency department physician, internist, thoracic surgeon
Urology	Anesthesiologist, internist, director of nursing, urologist

FIGURE 2.7

REAPPOINTMENT ACTIVITY SUMMARY

Appointee: _____ Date: _____ Years on staff: _____
Department affiliation: _____ Staff category: _____
Clinical privileges: _____

Activity profile

_____ Number of admissions   _____ Number of consults performed
_____ Number of surgical procedures _____ Number of consults ordered
_____ Number of invasive procedures

Membership information

Meeting attendance
Medical staff meetings   Attended _____ out of _____
Committee meetings (if any): Attended _____ out of _____
Departmental meetings   Attended _____ out of _____

Evidence of CME on file   ❏ Yes   ❏ No   Number of hours _____

Medical records completion
Number of times on suspension (if any): _____
Reappointment dues paid (if required)   ❏ Yes   ❏ No
License and DEA number verified   ❏ Yes   ❏ No
National Practitioner Data Bank report received   ❏ Yes   ❏ No
Professional liability insurance verified   ❏ Yes   ❏ No
Any OIG or state sanctions   ❏ Yes* ❏ No
Any known felony criminal actions   ❏ Yes* ❏ No
Any patient/staff complaints   ❏ Yes* ❏ No

*Please explain: _____

Clinical profile

Gross data
Overall mortality rate: _____ Average length of stay: _____
Number of autopsies ordered: _____
Disciplinary action (previous two years): _____
Number of documented patient complaints: _____
Number of malpractice claims filed: _____

Note: *Attach the physician profile/report to this form along with a summary of pertinent quality assurance/ improvement data.*

FIGURE 2.7

REAPPOINTMENT ACTIVITY SUMMARY (CONT.)

Gynecology monitoring   Number of charts reviewed: _____

Indicator number	1	2	3	4	5	6	7	8	9	10	11	12	13	14	15	16
Number of variations																
Departmental average																

Medical monitoring   Number of charts reviewed: _____

Indicator number	1	2	3	4	5	6	7	8	9	10	11	12	13	14	15	16
Number of variations																
Departmental average																

Pediatric monitoring   Number of charts reviewed: _____

Indicator number	1	2	3	4	5	6	7	8	9	10	11	12	13	14	15	16
Number of variations																
Departmental average																

Surgical monitoring   Number of charts reviewed: _____

Indicator number	1	2	3	4	5	6	7	8	9	10	11	12	13	14	15	16
Number of variations																
Departmental average																

Summary of findings from medical staff review activities

(Note presence or absence of significant problems identified through review activity.)

Surgical case review: _____

Antibiotic and drug use review: _____

Blood use review: _____

Special care unit care review: _____

Mortality review: _____

Utilization review: _____

Medical records review: _____

Departmental review: _____

FIGURE 2.8 — FAST-TRACK CREDENTIALING POLICY

It is this hospital's policy to process all applications only after the medical staff office receives a completed, verified application. It is the intent of this policy to expedite applications that meet predefined, board-approved criteria.

FAST-TRACK PROCEDURE

The credentials chair and medical staff services coordinator will review each application and its associated additional information, and will categorize the application according to the following criteria:

Category One
A. The applicant promptly returns all requested information

B. There are no negative or questionable recommendations

C. There are no discrepancies in information received from the applicant or references

D. The applicant completed a normal education/training sequence

E. There are no reports of disciplinary actions or legal sanctions

F. There are no reports of malpractice cases within the past two years

G. The applicant has an unremarkable medical staff/employment history

H. The applicant submits a reasonable request for clinical privileges based on experience, training, and competence and is in compliance with applicable criteria

I. The applicant reports an acceptable health status

J. The applicant has never had third-party payer (e.g., Medicare, Medicaid, etc.) sanctions

K. The applicant has no felony convictions

L. The applicant's history shows an ability to relate to others in a harmonious, collegial manner

Category Two
A. Peer references and/or prior affiliations indicate potential problems (e.g., difficulty with interpersonal relationships, minor patient care issues, etc.)

B. There are discrepancies between information the applicant submitted and information received from other sources

C. The applicant requests privileges that vary from those requested by other practitioners in the same specialty

D. The application includes unaccounted-for gaps in time

E. There are unsatisfactory peer references and/or prior affiliation references

F. A state licensing board or a state or federal regulatory agency took disciplinary action against the applicant, or the applicant has had a criminal conviction

G. The applicant has experienced voluntary or involuntary termination of medical staff membership, or voluntary or involuntary limitation, reduction, or loss of clinical privileges at another health care organization

FIGURE
2.8

FAST-TRACK CREDENTIALING POLICY (CONT.)

H. The applicant no longer serves on a provider panel of a managed care entity for reasons of unprofessional conduct or quality-of-care issues

I. The applicant has been the object of three or more malpractice claims/settlements/judgments in the past five years

J. The applicant has held a substantial number (more than five) of medical licenses across the United States

K. The applicant has had many healthcare organization affiliations in multiple areas during the past five years

PROCEDURE FOR PROCESSING CATEGORIES ONE AND TWO APPLICATIONS

Category One

1. The medical staff office receives and processes the application.

2. The appropriate department chair (and credentials chair) reviews the completed and verified application and all supporting materials.

   Note: *The credentials chair could be omitted if department chair review is acceptable and there are no problems noted.*

3. The department chair (and credentials chair) forwards a report with findings and a recommendation to the medical executive committee (MEC).

   The provisions of the medical staff bylaws must be followed to constitute an official MEC meeting. The Joint Commission on Accreditation of Healthcare Organizations (JCAHO) does not dictate quorum requirements. Therefore, the medical staff can specify that the MEC may meet for official business when a quorum of three members is present. These members could include the president of the staff, applicable department chair, and chief executive officer (CEO). The board may designate this group as a board subcommittee and empower it to act on all medical staff applications for appointment and clinical privileges. Such authority should be subject to the submission of minutes to the board for formal approval. The board should reserve the authority for all denials or revocations.

4. The medical staff president then forwards the MEC's recommendation to the board's authorized subcommittee, which (pursuant to a policy adopted by the board) grants the applicant appointment to the staff and the requested clinical privileges.

   Note: *The board subcommittee must be composed of at least two board members (e.g. CEO, chief of staff, or chair of the board).*

FIGURE
2.8

FAST-TRACK CREDENTIALING POLICY (CONT.)

---

5. The board's subcommittee makes an informational report to the board at its next regular meeting. The board does not take any action, as the hospital's bylaws or policy allow the board's subcommittee to act on the board's behalf in granting appointment and clinical privileges to any Category One physician agreed upon by the department chair, credentials committee chair, and MEC.

   Note: *If the department chair's recommendation is negative or differs from that of the credentials committee chair or MEC, the application is automatically classified as Category Two and processed accordingly.*

Category Two

1. The application is forwarded to the appropriate department chair for review and recommendation. The department chair reviews the application to ensure that it meets the established standards for membership and clinical privileges.

2. The department chair forwards the application to the credentials committee for review and recommendation. The credentials committee reviews the application for membership and clinical privileges.

3. The credentials committee then forwards the application to the MEC president for review and recommendation.

4. The MEC forwards the application with its recommendation to the board for final action.

   Note: *In the event the MEC's recommendation is negative, the hospital must review and follow its fair hearing plan.*

5. The MEC prepares a report for the board that identifies those practitioners who were appointed and granted clinical privileges via this mechanism.

GUIDELINES FOR RESPONDING TO LOW- AND NO-VOLUME PRACTITIONERS' APPLICATIONS

Your organization should use the appraisal/reappraisal process discussed in the previous chapter as a guide when processing a low- or no-volume provider's medical staff appointment/clinical privileges request.

The appraisal/reappraisal process detailed in Chapter two is built on the principle that all practitioners who request medical staff membership/clinical privileges must provide the hospital with evidence of current clinical competence. Remember, competency is the main issue when appointing and reappointing a physician to the medical staff and when granting or modifying a physician's clinical privileges. This is true whether the physician is an active member of the medical staff or a low- or no-volume provider.

Whenever privileges are involved, competency must be demonstrated.

The first steps

A hospital that must assess the competency of a low- or no-volume practitioner should first determine whether he or she actively practices at another accredited healthcare facility—step eight of the appraisal/reappraisal process outlined in the previous chapter.

Step nine of the appraisal/reappraisal process specifies that the hospital must determine whether the provider performs satisfactory clinical work at another organization.

To answer this question, the medical staff office (MSO) must collect volume and performance data from the facility at which the practitioner actively practices.

If the physician provides care at another accredited healthcare facility, your job of assessing his or her competency is conceptually quite easy. Your credentials committee can turn to that organization for evidence of the physician's competency. However, your hospital may have trouble obtaining from that organization information needed to assess the practitioner's competency. Remember, if that facility is reluctant to release the information, you must put the burden on the applicant.

You may discover that the practitioner applicant does not actively practice at another inpatient facility but rather focuses his or her practice on treating patients in an ambulatory setting. If this is the case, your task of evaluating requests for medical staff appointment is again fairly straightforward but, assessing the physician's request for clinical privileges may be daunting.

Your task remains the same in this situation—you must determine what information the organization needs to assess whether the physician is competent to perform the requested privileges. You must then decide the best course for obtaining that information.

Tip: Before processing the physician's request for privileges, hospital and medical staff leaders should engage in a collegial conversation with the physician applicant to determine whether he or she is interested in privileges that authorize him or her to treat patients on an inpatient basis.

In many instances, physicians who practice only in the ambulatory setting are satisfied with medical staff appointment and have no interest in obtaining inpatient treatment privileges (see Chapter four for information about separating issues of medical staff appointment from those of clinical privileges). Suggest to the physician that dependent privileges or privileges to "refer and follow" may be the best options.

"Refer and follow" privileges are often granted to physicians with busy office practices. These privileges allow the physician only to refer patients to the hospital. The provider can follow the patient's progress, but the attending physician at the hospital provides the necessary patient care. Most low- and no-volume physicians agree to this option because it allows them to demonstrate to managed care organizations that they have the ability to admit patients to the hospital when needed.

Because such physicians are not exercising hospital privileges anyway, most are happy to accept referral privileges, maintain medical staff membership, and continue to serve on committees, use the library, and attend medical staff meetings.

When processing applications submitted by physicians who simply refer patients to your hospital for treatment, you do not have to determine their competence to treat myocardial infarction, strokes, obstetrics, pneumonia, etc., because the physician is not requesting privileges to treat such cases. The physician is only requesting the privilege to admit his or her patients to your facility when necessary.

Lastly, consider the physician who is not clinically active at any facility. When faced with an appointment or clinical privileges request submitted by such physicians, an entirely different set of issues arises. Hospitals should never grant independent clinical privileges to such practitioners.

It can be difficult to process medical staff and privileging requests submitted by physicians who meet the above descriptions. For guidance through the process, consider the basic credentialing rules discussed in the next section of this book.

Basic credentialing rules

When faced with a membership application or clinical privilege request submitted by a low- or no-volume practitioner, turn to the following basic credentialing rules to decide how best to process that request:

1. Put the burden on the practitioner

Some hospitals spend too much time verifying credentials and reviewing requests for privileges, especially when handling requests made by low- or no-volume providers. Don't spend days making telephone calls and sending letters to the same institutions and individuals requesting information about an applicant.

If you are unable to obtain information about the practitioner from primary or reliable secondary sources, put the burden on the practitioner to gather the necessary information.

Remember, no hospital or organization should appoint a practitioner to the medical staff or grant him or her clinical privileges until it receives, verifies, and evaluates all required information. There is no exception to this rule.

Send an appropriately drafted business letter to the practitioner informing him or her that the MSO will terminate the appointment, reappointment, and/or privileging process if references fail to respond, if another organization fails to confirm affiliations and disciplinary information, or if another facility is reluctant to provide needed peer review information.

In many cases, the information source will be more responsive to the practitioner's request than to the hospital's request. See **Figure 3.0** on p. 65 for a sample burden on the practitioner policy.

For guidance on how to request additional information/clarification from a medical staff applicant, take a look at the instructions in **Figure 3.1** on p. 66. Turn to **Figure 3.2** on p. 67 for a sample letter to notify an applicant of an incomplete application.

Because the termination of the medical staff application process can be a controversial step, consider using the sample letters shown in **Figures 3.3** and **3.4** on pp. 68 and 69 to solicit additional information from an applicant before withdrawing his or her application.

2. The competency equation must be met

The competency equation asks what the provider has done and whether he or she has done it well. You must answer these questions before you can confidently approve a practitioner's request for medical staff membership/privileges.

This competency information is vital because appointment, reappointment, and privileging decisions are only as good as the available information.

Credentials committees and medical executive committees (MECs) should be vigilant about obtaining and reviewing clinical outcomes measures and reliable professional references to get an accurate picture of a physician's current clinical competence.

To meet the competency equation, a department chair must determine that the low-or no-volume practitioner is engaged in relevant recent clinical work at either your hospital or another accredited facility. Ensure that the practitioner's work meets your quality standards.

If a practitioner is active at another facility, accreditation and regulatory agencies' regulations require hospitals to obtain information that details the clinical work the practitioner performs at that institution. In addition, you must receive confirmation from knowledgeable sources at that facility that the quality of the practitioner's work is acceptable, and that the practitioner complies with applicable policies and procedures regarding patient care and professional behavior. This task also takes place during step nine of the appraisal/reappraisal process detailed in Chapter two.

3. Other institutions are not obligated to respond

There are no laws or regulations that compel an institution to provide another facility with information about a member of its medical staff. However, hospitals have long relied on each other to comply voluntarily with reasonable requests to furnish information concerning a practitioner's clinical volume and quality of care.

If an institution refuses to provide requested information, the burden for producing that information must be placed on the practitioner applying for membership/privileges. Occasionally, neither the facility nor the physician has access to the requested information. When this situation arises, the credentialing professional or department chair should simply inform the physician that the hospital will cease processing his or her application until the needed data is submitted for review.

4. Simply because there is no reason to deny or reject is not a reason to approve requests for clinical privileges

Medical staff leaders must resolve any and all doubts about an applicant's or reapplicant's past experience, education, training, references, health status, behavior, citizenship, etc.

If the credentials committee or MEC has any reservations, however small, about any aspect of a physician's background or current clinical competence, it should investigate further and gather information necessary to proceed confidently with the appointment/privileging process.

In many instances, a low- or no-volume practitioner will submit a credentials file that is free of red flags. However, a problem-free file is not reason enough to recommend medical staff appointment or grant clinical privileges. As stated earlier in this chapter, the file must contain evidence of the practitioner's current clinical competence before granting privileges.

5. Do not confuse appointment to the staff, a category, or a department with the granting of clinical privileges

See Chapter four for more information about separating requests for medical staff membership from requests for clinical privilege.

6. Reappointment of a practitioner who no longer engages in significant clinical activity at the hospital depends on the evaluation of the physician's general qualifications.

These qualifications include

- licensure
- malpractice history
- disciplinary actions taken by other agencies and healthcare organizations
- databank information
- criminal history
- Medicaid and Medicare sanctions
- general adherence to professional ethics and professional standards

These factors are, after all, what we usually evaluate when reappointing a dentist, dermatologist, or allergist who infrequently uses the hospital's resources. Although these practitioners have few or no patient contacts at the hospital, the hospital's medical staff and credentialing professionals manage to determine whether they qualify for reappointment. The hospital finds a place for these physicians on the medical staff because they are good practitioners and active members of the community.

However, a different set of challenges arises when considering current clinical competence and privileges. The hospital cannot simply grant a physician the privilege to refer patients to the facility without evidence that he or she is a competent practitioner. The hospital has no interest in appointing to its medical staff a practitioner with a poor professional reputation.

Therefore, insist on at least one or two letters or questionnaires of recommendation from physicians on your medical staff to whom the physician applicant refers patients. These recommendations could come from a hospitalist and at least one other physician who knows of the general professional performance and reputation of the nonadmitting physician.

With these basic credentialing rules in mind, set aside time to review your current credentialing processes and procedures. You may have to adjust your credentialing systems to

- ensure a clear separation of appointment and privileging issues
- develop a new questionnaire to gather professional recommendations for nonactive physicians
- make it clear that clinical privileges to admit and treat patients at your facility depends on the practitioner's ability to demonstrate specific current clinical competence in acute care provided in a complex hospital environment

Remember, these changes generally do not require your hospital to make changes to its medical staff bylaws. They only require a change in the organization's mindset.

Note: Turn to **Figure 3.5** on p. 70 for a list of appointment and clinical privileges myths and truths.

FIGURE 3.0

SAMPLE POLICY AND PROCEDURE: PLACING THE BURDEN ON THE APPLICANT

Policy

Each individual practitioner who either applies for or maintains medical staff membership and/or privileges has the burden of providing evidence that demonstrates, in the sole discretion of the hospital, that he or she meets the hospital's established criteria for membership and privileges. This policy applies at the time of initial appointment, reappointment, application for clinical privileges, employment, or at any time during a practitioner's affiliation with the institution.

Procedure

In order to fulfill this responsibility, the practitioner has the burden of producing any information requested by the hospital or its authorized representatives that is reasonably necessary, in the sole discretion of the hospital, to evaluate whether or not the practitioner meets the criteria for medical staff membership and privileges.

If there is undo delay in obtaining such required information or if the hospital requires clarification of such information, the medical staff office will request the applicant's assistance (see sample letter, p. 68. Under these circumstances, the medical staff may modify its usual and customary time periods for processing the application or reapplication. The hospital has sole discretion for determining what is an adequate response.

If, during the process of initial application or reapplication, the applicant fails to respond adequately within 30 days to a request for information or assistance, the hospital will deem the application or reapplication as being withdrawn voluntarily (see sample notification letter, p. 69). The result of the withdrawal is automatic termination of the application or reapplication process. The hospital will not consider the termination an adverse action. Therefore, the applicant or reapplicant is not entitled to a fair hearing or appeal consistent with the medical staff's fair hearing plan. The hospital will not report the action to any external agency.

| FIGURE 3.1 | INSTRUCTIONS FOR REQUESTING ADDITIONAL INFORMATION/CLARIFICATION |

Once your hospital receives a complete application for medical staff appointment, it is obligated to process that application according to the timeframes outlined in your medical staff bylaws. However, a practitioner's failure to submit a complete application does affect the time frame for processing his or her application. It's important that you clearly document and follow up on requests you send to an applicant for more additional information.

The hospital must promptly notify the applicant when more information or clarification is needed before his or her application can be processed. This request should be made in writing and sent by certified mail. The letter should

- specify the information needed
- make clear the time frame within which the applicant must submit the information
- inform the applicant that his or her lack of response to the request will result in the voluntary withdrawal of the application

The medical staff office must then

- file a copy of all related correspondence in the credentials file
- document the information sent and received in the master control log
- track the time frames for receipt of the requested information
- withdraw the application from process if the applicant does not respond to the request
- contact the applicant regarding receipt, unsatisfactory response, or non-receipt

---

FIGURE 3.2

NOTIFICATION OF INCOMPLETE APPLICATION

[*Date*]

Dear [*name*]:

We have received your application for medical staff appointment request for clinical privileges at [*hospital name*].

However, our initial review of your application and the request for clinical privileges determined that additional information and/or clarification is necessary before we can continue processing your application. I have detailed the needed information and/or clarification in an attachment to this letter.

Please send a written response to this request, including all requested information, to my attention. Your response should be sent no later than [*date*].

We will resume processing your application once we receive a satisfactory reply from you. If we do not receive a reply by the date noted above, your application will be considered voluntarily withdrawn and your file will be closed.

Thank you for your cooperation in this matter.

Sincerely,

[*Manager, credentialing services*]

Enclosures

NOTIFICATION OF UNSATISFACTORY RESPONSE

[*Date*]

Dear [*name*],

Thank you for your response to my letter dated [*date*], which requested additional information and/or clarification of information in your application for medical staff appointment and clinical privileges. However, we have reviewed your response and determined that we require further information and/or clarification of information.

I have attached a separate document to this letter that explains why your reply was deemed non-responsive, and specifies what information you must provide to adequately respond to our request.

Please submit accurate, complete information in response to this inquiry at your earliest convenience. Your written response must be sent no later than [*date*].

We will resume processing your application once we receive a satisfactory reply from you. If we do not receive a reply by the date noted above, your application will be considered voluntarily withdrawn and your file will be closed.

Thank you for your cooperation in this matter.

Sincerely,

[*Chief operating officer*]

Enclosures

FIGURE
3.4

NOTIFICATION OF FAILURE TO RESPOND

[*Date*]

Dear [*name*]:

In the letter dated [*date of first notification*], we notified you that we required additional information or clarification to process your application for appointment to the medical staff and/or your request for specific clinical privileges. We also informed you your application would be considered voluntarily withdrawn if we did not receive a reply by the date specified.

Therefore, we view your failure to reply to our request before that date as an indication that you wish to withdraw your application. Accordingly, we have terminated a review of the application and closed your file. We may reopen your file if you complete a new application that includes the information missing from your initial application, and an explanation for your failure to respond to our request for additional information. If you submit a second application, you must include the full amount of the application fee. We will process your second application in the same manner as all initial applications for medical staff membership.

If extenuating circumstances prevented you from responding to our request before the deadline, please provide us with a written explanation of those circumstances. Such explanations should be sent to my attention by [reply date] along with the additional information or clarification originally requested. If this explanation is found satisfactory by the hospital and medical staff leaders, we will resume processing your application.

Thank you for your cooperation in this matter.

Sincerely,

[*President and Chief operating officer*]

```
┌─────────────────────────────────────────────────────────────────────────────┐
```

FIGURE 3.5   APPOINTMENT AND CLINICAL PRIVILEGES
                                                              MYTHS AND TRUTHS

Myth: Privileges are owned by the physician.

Truth: Privileges are short-term grants made by the hospital's governing board. Such grants generally expire within 24 months. Practitioners must reapply if they are interested in another grant of the same or modified privileges.

Myth: Denials of requests for clinical privileges are always reportable to the National Practitioner Data Bank (NPDB).

Truth: Denials of requested privileges due to the physician's failure to meet the institution's threshold criteria—inadequate education, training, or experience—are not reportable to the NPDB.

Myth: Assignment to the active category requires that the physician be regularly involved in the care of hospitalized patients.

Truth: Medical staff bylaws may define any qualification for assignment to the active category. For example, bylaws may state that assignment to the active category requires the physician to demonstrate an interest in assisting the hospital and medical staff in meeting its patient care mission.

The physician may demonstrate his or her commitment to the patient care mission by providing evidence of his or her admissions, procedures, referrals; work on medical staff or board committees; service at the facility's free clinic; or participation as an instructor in the facility's continuing education program.

Myth: Requests for continued clinical privileges should always be granted unless there is evidence that demonstrates that the physician is not competent to provide such patient care services.

Truth: Privileges should never be granted unless there is compelling evidence demonstrating that the physician is currently competent to provide such services.

| FIGURE 3.5 | APPOINTMENT AND CLINICAL PRIVILEGES MYTHS AND TRUTHS (CONT.) |

Myth: Any time a physician's privileges are not renewed (at reappointment) the physician is entitled to a fair hearing.

Truth: Fair hearings are held if the medical executive committee or board takes action to revoke or deny a request for privileges due to concerns about the physician's performance. Hearings are not designed for instances in which a physician's privileges have expired and are not renewed due to the absence of recent relevant clinical experience.

Myth: Managed care organizations (MCOs) require that physicians with whom they contract hold clinical privileges at an accredited hospital.

Truth: Most MCOs no longer require physicians to have clinical privileges at a hospital. At one time, MCOs did not conduct physician performance evaluations or credentialing. They required physician to hold medical staff membership and clinical privileges to ensure that they were qualified. In essence, the MCO was piggybacking on the hospital's credentials program. However, the National Committee for Quality Assurance now requires accredited MCOs to conduct credentialing.

Myth: There is a direct correlation between incompetence and low- or no-volume of work performed by a physician.

Truth: Low- and no-volume of work may suggest that the practitioner is likely to have poorer outcomes than a high-volume physician. However, the lack of volume does not in and of itself indicate that the physician is incompetent. It simply means that there is little or no evidence for the hospital to analyze to determine whether the physician is competent.

OPTIONS FOR PROCESSING LOW- AND NO-VOLUME PROVIDERS' APPLICATIONS

When considering how best to process medical staff membership and clinical privileges requests submitted by low- and no-volume providers, the credentials committee and medical executive committee (MEC) should keep in mind the appraisal/reappraisal flowchart in Chapter two that depicts the application processing steps and decision points and the general guidelines discussed in Chapter three.

Following the steps outlined on the flowchart should help committee members navigate the options available and ensure the fair treatment of all practitioners applying for membership/clinical privileges.

The process is determined by the individual practitioner

The approach you take to gathering evidence of a low- or no-volume practitioner's competence depends on the reason for which the practitioner performs few or no clinical procedures at your organization.

The following physicians are typical low- and no-volume applicants:

①The provider treats the majority or all of his or her patients at another facility.
In such instances, the job of assessing the practitioner's competence is not very difficult. If the low- or no-volume practitioner has significant clinical activity at another facility—e.g., ambulatory care center, surgicenter, or hospital—send a questionnaire to responsible individuals at that site seeking confirmation of the practitioner's clinical knowledge, technical skill, professional performance, absence of disciplinary

issues, judgment, behavior, and any additional factors relevant to clinical privileging decisions.

Obtain references from that hospital's chief executive officer, department chair, and director of medical records. See **Figure 4.1** on p. 86 for a sample letter that should accompany the reference questionnaire. See **Figure 4.2** on p. 87 for a sample professional reference questionnaire.

Collect volume and outcomes data from the other institution. To gather this information, put the burden on the physician applying for privileges. The physician should ensure the provision of

- his or her volume of clinical activity at the facility
- confirmation of medical staff status "in good standing" with no disciplinary actions, no contemplated investigations, and no ongoing investigations or quality/peer review adverse actions
- confirmation from the relevant department chair that the physician is clinically competent in all areas covered by his or her requested privileges

②The physician is not clinically active at another institution but is active within the community (e.g., is a family physician, dermatologist, or allergist).
If a low- or no-volume volume practitioner is not active at another facility but remains active at an ambulatory facility or at his or her own office, current clinical competence can be gathered using the following mechanisms:

- The low- or no-volume practitioner should produce a specified number of patient records that reflects his or her clinical work.

Your credentials committee can opt to appoint a member of your medical staff to review the work the provider has done in his or her office that is comparable to procedures performed at the hospital. The hospital may require the physician applying for privileges to compensate the physician who conducts the review. However, many hospitals share this expense equally with the physician.

You can also appoint an outside expert to review the physician's patient records. Hospitals typically choose this option when the practitioner applicant directly competes with a current member of the medical staff who would normally be responsible for the review and evaluation of the applicant's practice.

A review of patient records (properly edited to comply with the Health Insurance Portability and Accountability Act of 1996) will show whether the physician ordered the right ancillaries, made appropriate and timely consults, and documented legibly.

- The low- or no-volume practitioner should provide three physician references who have worked with him or her and who can attest to his or her skills, knowledge, ability, technique, and ability to get along with patients. Physicians who refer to the practitioner and are able to assess the results of the referral are good candidates for providing references.

The general rule is that only individuals who know and agree to report on the adequacy of the physician's clinical work in his or her private office should complete the reference questionnaire. These three references must provide documentation that shows what the physician has done and that he or she has done it well.

- The low- or no-volume physician should provide your credentials committee with a billing printout of procedures performed in his or her office. The billing information should include information about the volume and type of procedures.

The official billing printout will allow the chairs of the MEC and credentials committee to comfortably recommend the physician for level one privileges.

- Your hospital can also collect performance data by consulting the physician's "report card," put together by his or her managed care organization, and conducting a survey of procedures performed by the physician in his or her office.

③The physician has not practiced medicine for several years

A physician's extended absence from medicine presents additional challenges. It is unacceptable to grant independent clinical privileges to such practitioners, but do not shut these physicians out of your hospital. Your organization should a have policy to allow these physicians to reenter medicine.

For example, you can require the physician to co-admit his or her patients, work in conjunction with a senior physician, work with a proctor, or complete a mini or full residency.

It is virtually impossible to assess the current clinical competency of a low- or no-volume practitioner who is not active in any clinical setting. Therefore, it is necessary to observe his or her clinical work directly in a highly controlled environment.

In general, physicians with no current clinical activity should be granted clinical privileges only if they agree to proctoring or observation. These physicians are good candidates for dependent clinical privileges, which permit them to provide specified patient care services only in conjunction with a qualified, clinically active, competent practitioner.

At the conclusion of a specified period of time, the department chair can rely on assessments and information provided by the physicians co-treating patients with the low- or no-volume practitioner to make clinical privileging decisions.

Review your organization's proctoring policy and associated forms to ensure that they capture the competency data you need to confidently grant a practitioner full privileges. Turn to **Figure 4.3** on p. 90 for a sample proctoring guidelines. Turn to **Figure 4.4** on p. 93 for a sample proctor assignment procedure.

Separate medical staff membership from clinical privileges

When faced with an initial application or reapplication submitted by a low- or no-volume provider, remember to separate the issue of medical staff membership from that of clinical privileges.

Remember, the term credentialing refers to the overall process of gathering and verifying credentials information, reviewing that information, and making a decision to grant or deny medical staff membership. Although both appointment to the medical staff and granting of clinical privileges are part of the credentialing process, they are not one and the same.

Medical staff membership only allows physicians access to the physicians' dining room, hospital library, continuing medical education classes, and voting rights, if allowed by hospital policy. In addition, granting membership allows the physician to advertise his or her affiliation with your organization and satisfy managed care organizations' requirements.

Physicians who only seek medical staff appointment should complete an application or reapplication form, submit letters or completed reference questionnaires from colleagues, and provide a description of his or her private practice or practice at another facility. The hospital should also require the physician to complete an intended practice plan (IPP). Turn to **Figure 4.5** on p. 95 for a sample IPP.

Remember, appointing a physician to your medical staff does not automatically allow him or her to treat patients. Therefore, your credentials committee can recommend medical staff membership for a low- or no-volume provider who desires affiliation with your hospital but who does not want or need privileges to admit and treat patients.

If your organization wants the option of granting membership without privileges, the hospital's policy must allow you to take that route. For example, if your hospital's membership criteria require members to provide emergency department on-call coverage, your organization will not have the option of appointing a physician to the medical staff without also granting privileges.

Under such circumstances, inform the provider that he or she does not meet your organization's minimum criteria for membership and the MSO will therefore not process the application.

Tip: Your credentials committee and MEC must recommend membership criteria to the governing board before applying them to a medical staff applicant. Once the board approves the criteria, write them into the medical staff bylaws and policies.

Example: Membership without privileges

The decision to grant a physician medical staff membership without clinical privileges traditionally is made when appointing a physician to the honorary or emeritus staff. It is logical to extend this principle to include physicians whose practice is directly supportive of the hospital's mission but who do not perform any clinical work in or under the auspice of the hospital.

For example, a family physician with an active office-based practice supports the hospital's mission by directing all of his or her patients to the institution's hospitalist program or staff consultants for inpatient treatment. The physician also directs all of his patients in need of emergency care to the hospital and relies on the facility's outpatient services for particular tests and therapy (e.g., radiology, physical therapy, and occupational therapy).

The MSO could easily process this physician's request for membership on the active medical staff and privileges to "refer and follow" (see Chapter three for more information about "refer and follow" privileges.)

The MSO should gather information demonstrating the physician's compliance with basic appointment criteria set out by the medical staff bylaws. The physician's colleagues should submit one or two letters that confirm that the physician is in good standing in the medical community. This information would allow the credentials committee to determine that the physician's medical staff appointment would not jeopardize the hospital's or medical staff's reputation in the community.

Appointment to the medical staff would allow the physician access to nonclinical rights of active staff status and assignment to the department of primary care. As mentioned previously, medical staff appointment may also allow the physician to vote, hold office, chair committees, advise management and the board, and participate in other medical staff activities.

However, the organization's medical staff bylaws may prohibit the physician from joining the hospital's active medical staff. Traditional medical staff bylaws often prevent credentialing and medical staff professionals from effectively processing medical staff membership requests made by low- and no-volume practitioners by requiring that practitioners on the active medical staff perform many procedures at the facility. They also require the physician to receive referrals from the emergency department or participate in medical staff affairs.

In addition, traditional bylaws often state that a physician must be on the active staff at another facility for the hospital to grant him or her courtesy appointment. This requirement is designed to ensure that all physicians are subject to at least one medical staff's peer review process and that they are required to fulfill medical staff responsibilities.

Further, appointment to the provisional category is most often reserved for new applicants. Traditional bylaws require these individuals to provide care in the hospital to allow the medical staff to observe their initial work before deciding whether to appoint them to the active or courtesy staff category.

These bylaws fail to recognize that many providers—allergists, dermatologists, family physicians, surgeons, and a few other specialists—now find it unnecessary to rely on hospital resources even though they remain an invaluable component of the healthcare delivery system. Bylaws that insist that these practitioners maintain active staff appointment fail to recognize changes in the delivery of healthcare.

Your bylaws should allow such physicians to join the associate or affiliate staff. The bylaws should detail the responsibilities of practitioners appointed to these staff categories. See **Figure 4.6** on p. 97 for sample bylaws language.

If you decide to grant a physician membership without privileges, you are not obligated to confirm the physician's specific clinical competence because the practitioner does not seek to exercise privileges at the organization. All of his or her patients in need of acute hospital services would receive those services through direct referral by this physician to other medical staff members with clinical privileges. Make sure that your credentialing policies and procedures note this option.

If the physician wishes to maintain clinical privileges that allow him or her to actively treat acutely ill patients, he or she must provide evidence that demonstrates current clinical competence. In short, he or she must ensure that the competency equation is met to the satisfaction of the department chair and credentials committee. However, the physician in question may have difficulty providing this information because he or she has not recently provided care to acutely ill patients and is therefore unable to demonstrate inpatient performance results. Some credentials committees would have significant difficulty if faced with this dilemma.

Note: When a practitioner seeks clinical privileges for authorization to treat acutely ill patients but cannot provide evidence demonstrating the skills necessary to provide such treatment, it is not the credentials committee's responsibility to prove that the physician is incompetent. It is the practitioner's responsibility to furnish evidence demonstrating that he or she meets the minimum threshold criteria established by the medical staff for inpatient privileges.

Additional options: Modifying requests, denials

Credentials committees are permitted, when necessary, to request that a practitioner modify his or her request for clinical privileges. This option is particularly important when there is a chance that the practitioner's privileging request may be formally denied.

Most experienced credentialing professionals recognize the importance of avoiding denials and use other techniques to ensure that quality patient care is delivered in a safe environment.

Department chairs should not hesitate to alert the credentials committee and MEC when they are unable to assess current clinical competence due to the absence of information, as noted in step 22 of the appraisal/reappraisal process discussed in Chapter two. The credentials committee or MEC must then use their experience, skills, and knowledge to appropriately respond to this unusual circumstance. Such situations typically arise when a practitioner chooses a practice style that does not require him or her to work at the facility.

Course of action

Now that we've established what a low- and no-volume provider is, discussed the traditional appraisal and reappraisal process, and presented strategies for assessing the competency of low- and no-volume providers, we will discuss a few scenarios that will help guide your response to medical staff membership and privileging requests made by low- and no-volume practitioners.

Nearly all medical staffs recognize that it would be illogical to grant a board-certified cardiothoracic surgeon clinical privileges if he or she has not worked in the operating room for two years. In fact, many medical staffs would not be comfortable recommending this physician for any surgical privileges.

However, some medical staffs might opt to recommend privileges for this individual if he or she agrees to exercise those privileges only in conjunction with a fully qualified cardiothoracic surgeon on the medical staff.

Likewise, a medical staff would likely tell an anesthesiologist who has not provided anesthesia in a hospital or organized surgicenter in the past two years that he or she does not qualify for anesthesia privileges. The MSO may inform the anesthesiologist that he or she will have to participate in a retraining program to qualify for appointment. It is logical to extend this principle to general internists, family physicians, pediatricians, and other practitioners with active outpatient practices but no inpatient practices.

The medical staff's rules and regulations ideally would provide guidance in all of these areas. Unfortunately, many medical staffs have not permitted their rules and regulations to evolve and allow them to handle adequately these new circumstances.

Keep in mind the basic credentialing rules, appointment myths and truths, and lessons discussed earlier in this chapter when considering the following examples of low- and no-volume practitioners. In addition, remember the general principle that requires hospitals to grant privileges only after reviewing data that attests to the physician's current clinical competence.

The scenario: An excellent physician who has chosen to provide care only in the ambulatory setting has requested inpatient treatment privileges.

Upon receipt of requests for inpatient treatment privileges by the "nonactive physician," the hospital informs the physician that it can not process the request until the physician provides evidence demonstrating that he or she meets the organization's minimum threshold criteria established by the staff for the granting of such privileges.

The minimum threshold criteria require evidence that the physician provided inpatient care to acutely ill patients during the past two years, and that the physician's peers believe his or her work in this area to be of high quality.

The practitioner then must submit additional information as evidence that he or she is competent to perform the requested privileges. The department chair reviews the information to determine whether the organization should grant the physician privileges.

The steps your organization takes at this point in the process depends on the individual practitioner. For example, imagine that the physician requesting privileges is one of the following:

1. A retired plastic surgeon who is a current medical staff member

At the time of his reappointment, the provider requests full plastic surgical privileges. The department chair's review of the practitioner's clinical activity demonstrates that he does not have an active office practice and has not exercised privileges at any other facility.

In this case, the credentials committee should not hesitate to inform the practitioner that he is not eligible for full clinical privileges. The committee can opt to authorize the physician to provide care in conjunction with another qualified plastic surgeon on the medical staff. Requiring the physician to work alongside another practitioner is the only way that the organization could directly evaluate the quality of his work.

Credentials committees often overanalyze such situations to avoid insulting or criticizing a colleague. However, the best course of action is to deal with this issue in a businesslike manner. Rely on your policies and procedures to avoid the appearance of impropriety.

2. **A general internist on the medical staff who maintains only an ambulatory practice, but who requests clinical privileges that authorize her to admit and treat acutely ill patients**

   Your organization could use one or more of the techniques outlined above to assess the current clinical competence of this practitioner's ambulatory work. However, the assessment would demonstrate only the quality of the practitioner's work in the ambulatory setting and would not likely permit the hospital to grant the physician independent clinical privileges that authorize him or her to treat acutely ill patients.

   Once again, the credentials committee should suggest that the practitioner modify her privileging requests and seek only privileges to admit and treat patients in conjunction with another practitioner on the medical staff.

3. **A general surgeon on staff with no (or limited) clinical activity who maintains a very active hospital-based practice at a facility in reasonable proximity**

   The hospital should submit precise questionnaires to the other facility to gather information that would allow it to assess the physician's current clinical competence. The hospital can grant the practitioner full clinical privileges if the completed questionnaire attests to the physician's skill, judgment, and professional performance.

4. **An otolaryngologist who is interested in securing continued privileges in this area, but who performs all clinical work in his own surgicenter**

   Once again, the practitioner must submit directly to the hospital patient records that reflect his office work. The hospital must then conduct an internal or external evaluation of the patient records.

Alternatively, the hospital can request that the practitioner make patient records and reports available for peer review within his facility. Once such a review is performed, assuming that this review confirmed excellent clinical performance, it would be easy for the department chair to complete a report reflecting his opinion of the physician's competence, judgment, and skill.

FIGURE 4.1 LETTER ACCOMPANYING PROFESSIONAL REFERENCE QUESTIONNAIRE

[*Date*]

Practitioner's name (including any other name(s) used): _____
Date of birth: _____

The above-named practitioner has applied for medical staff appointment and clinical privileges at [*hospital name*]. The applicant listed you as a reference.

Based on your personal knowledge of the applicant, we would appreciate your candid, written appraisal of him/her. The enclosed professional reference questionnaire encompasses clinical ability, ethical character, ability to work cooperatively with others, health status, and other information relevant to this practitioner's qualifications for appointment and privileges.

We appreciate your providing your knowledge of these matters with respect to the applicant, particularly anything that warrants caution in granting him/her appointment or particular clinical privileges. A copy of his/her request for clinical privileges is attached so that you may assess the appropriateness of the privileges for which he/she has applied.

A self-addressed envelope is enclosed for your convenience. Your prompt and full response will be appreciated. Also enclosed is a copy of a release and immunity statement executed by the practitioner in connection with the application. This signed statement constitutes consent to this inquiry and to your response and releases from liability any individual who provides the requested information to representatives of this hospital.

Thank you for your cooperation.

Sincerely,

[*Chief executive officer or Vice president of medical affairs*]

FIGURE
4.2

PROFESSIONAL REFERENCE QUESTIONNAIRE

Professional evaluation concerning [*applicant's full name, including any other name(s) used*]:

_____

Specialties: _____

Date of birth: _____

Reference provided by: _____

Please check the accuracy of this information, and change/complete as appropriate.

Field of practice: _____

Present professional position: _____

Day phone: _____

Please answer all questions based on your personal knowledge and direct observations. Your candidness will be greatly appreciated.

I. Relationship of reference source to applicant

1. How long have you known the applicant? _____

2. During what time period did you have the opportunity to directly observe the applicant's practice of medicine?

   _____

3 a. In what setting(s) and with what frequency did you observe the applicant (i.e., office, hospital, residency program, etc. or daily, weekly, monthly, infrequently)? _____

   _____

   b. Was your observation done in connection with any official professional title or position? ❏ Yes   ❏ No

      If so, please indicate title and organization: _____

   c. What was the applicant's title or position? _____

4. Were you previously, are you now, or are you about to become related to the applicant as family or through a professional partnership or financial association?   ❏ Yes   ❏ No

   If yes, please explain: _____
   _____
   _____

FIGURE
4.2

PROFESSIONAL REFERENCE QUESTIONNAIRE (CONT.)

II. Professional knowledge, skills, and attitude

If you do not have adequate knowledge to answer a particular question, please indicate "No information."

1. Please rate the following:	Above average	Average	Below average	No information
a. Basic medical/clinical knowledge	❑	❑	❑	❑
b. Knowledge in specialty	❑	❑	❑	❑
c. Technical skills	❑	❑	❑	❑
d. Clinical judgment	❑	❑	❑	❑
e. Availability and thoroughness in patient care	❑	❑	❑	❑

	Satisfactory	Unsatisfactory	No information
f. Appropriate and timely use of consultants	❑	❑	❑
g. Quality/appropriateness of patient care outcomes	❑	❑	❑
h. Appropriateness of resource use (i.e. necessary for admissions, procedures, LOS, tests, etc.)	❑	❑	❑
i. Clarity/completeness of medical records	❑	❑	❑
j. Medical record timeliness	❑	❑	❑
k. Legibility of records	❑	❑	❑
l. Participation in committees, leadership, etc.	❑	❑	❑
m. Verbal and written fluency in English	❑	❑	❑
n. Rapport with patients	❑	❑	❑
o. Ability to work with others	❑	❑	❑

2 a. My recommendation concerning the specific clinical privileges/services requested is as follows:
  ❑ Recommend for all requested   ❑ Not recommend certain privileges/services
  ❑ Limit certain privileges/services   ❑ Not recommend for any privileges/services

  b. Please explain any reservations or concerns regarding any specific privileges/services requested by the applicant.

3. Have you ever observed or been informed of any problems that the applicant has or had that have affected or could potentially affect his/her ability to exercise any or all of the privileges requested or to perform the duties of medical staff appointment?   ❑ Yes   ❑ No   ❑ No information
  If yes, please explain: _____
  _____

FIGURE 4.2	*PROFESSIONAL REFERENCE QUESTIONNAIRE (CONT.)*

4. To the best of your knowledge, has the applicant's license, clinical privileges, hospital appointment, affiliation with any healthcare organization, or other professional status ever been denied, challenged, investigated, terminated, reduced, not renewed, limited, withdrawn, suspended, revoked, modified, placed on probation, or voluntarily surrendered, or do you have knowledge of any such actions that are pending?

❏ Yes   ❏ No   ❏ No information

If yes, please explain: _____
_____
_____

5. Do you know of any malpractice action instituted or in process against the applicant?

❏ Yes   ❏ No   ❏ No information

If yes, please explain: _____
_____
_____

III. Summary

1. My recommendation concerning this practitioner's application for appointment/affiliation is as follows:

❏ Recommended   ❏ Recommended with reservation   ❏ Not recommended

2. Please use this section for any additional comments, information, or recommendations that may be relevant to our decision to grant appointment/affiliation or specific clinical privileges/services to the applicant.

Signature: _____ Date: _____

FIGURE
4.3
SAMPLE GUIDELINES FOR PROCTORING

I. What is proctoring?

Proctoring is a requirement for medical staff appointment. New members are appointed to the provisional staff upon presentation of adequate and appropriate credentials. Provisional practitioner advancement (to the active or courtesy staff category) only occurs upon completion of the prescribed proctoring period. Members of the active, affiliate, and courtesy staff who apply for new and additional privileges are also subject to proctoring as defined in these guidelines. Each department needs to individualize its proctoring program.

II. Purpose of proctoring

The purpose of proctoring is to ensure that provisional practitioners are competent in areas of requested privileges. Proctoring is an important part of the privileging process, because it involves both direct observation and assessment of the new staff member's clinical ability. The process of proctoring should assure the proctor, the department chair, the medical executive committee, and the governing body that the new provisional practitioner provides quality care. A well-established system of proctoring is the medical staff's safeguard to prevent compromising quality patient care.

III. Proctoring policy

A. Provisional practitioners shall undergo proctoring for a [twelve-month period]. Under exceptional circumstances, the credentials committee, upon recommendation of the department chair, may extend the period of proctoring. Proctoring begins when the provisional practitioner commences patient care activities.

B. The proctor shall perform proctoring responsibilities by direct observation, as well as by concurrent and retrospective review of the provisional practitioner's cases. The extent of review is determined by the department chair and should be consistent with the breadth of privileges requested. Proctoring reports must be sufficiently detailed to provide an accurate measure of general and specific competency in all categories of privileges requested.

C. There shall be a minimum of two proctors for each new staff member.

D. In the reports proctoring reports should include the following:

    1. List each case proctored by the patient identification number, type of case, or procedure.

    2. Submit each case within 24 hours of the observation.

    3. Include the proctor's judgment about the appropriateness of care rendered.

    4. Base judgment based on direct observation of performance. Retrospective evaluation may be used as a supplement to direct observation. It is recognized that direct observation of psychotherapy and other

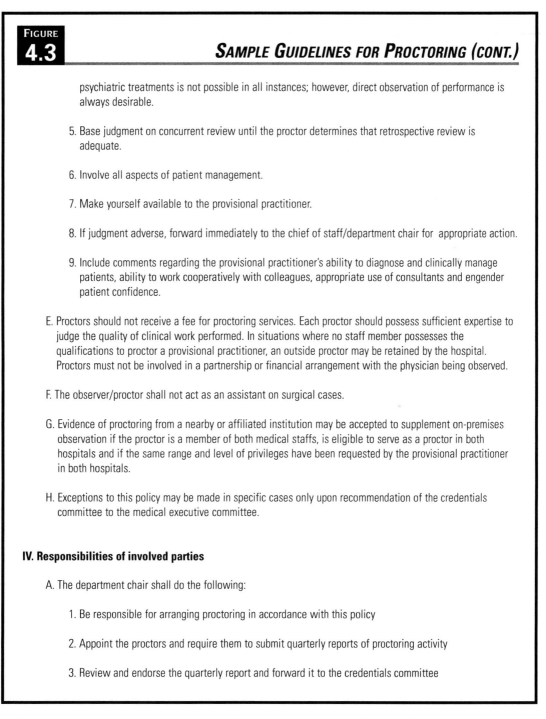

FIGURE 4.3

SAMPLE GUIDELINES FOR PROCTORING (CONT.)

psychiatric treatments is not possible in all instances; however, direct observation of performance is always desirable.

5. Base judgment on concurrent review until the proctor determines that retrospective review is adequate.

6. Involve all aspects of patient management.

7. Make yourself available to the provisional practitioner.

8. If judgment adverse, forward immediately to the chief of staff/department chair for appropriate action.

9. Include comments regarding the provisional practitioner's ability to diagnose and clinically manage patients, ability to work cooperatively with colleagues, appropriate use of consultants and engender patient confidence.

E. Proctors should not receive a fee for proctoring services. Each proctor should possess sufficient expertise to judge the quality of clinical work performed. In situations where no staff member possesses the qualifications to proctor a provisional practitioner, an outside proctor may be retained by the hospital. Proctors must not be involved in a partnership or financial arrangement with the physician being observed.

F. The observer/proctor shall not act as an assistant on surgical cases.

G. Evidence of proctoring from a nearby or affiliated institution may be accepted to supplement on-premises observation if the proctor is a member of both medical staffs, is eligible to serve as a proctor in both hospitals and if the same range and level of privileges have been requested by the provisional practitioner in both hospitals.

H. Exceptions to this policy may be made in specific cases only upon recommendation of the credentials committee to the medical executive committee.

IV. Responsibilities of involved parties

A. The department chair shall do the following:

1. Be responsible for arranging proctoring in accordance with this policy

2. Appoint the proctors and require them to submit quarterly reports of proctoring activity

3. Review and endorse the quarterly report and forward it to the credentials committee

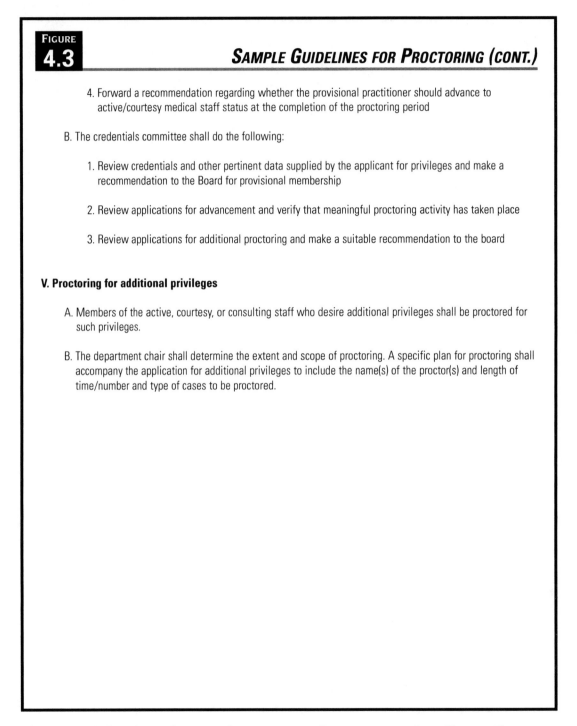

FIGURE
4.3

SAMPLE GUIDELINES FOR PROCTORING (CONT.)

  4. Forward a recommendation regarding whether the provisional practitioner should advance to active/courtesy medical staff status at the completion of the proctoring period

B. The credentials committee shall do the following:

  1. Review credentials and other pertinent data supplied by the applicant for privileges and make a recommendation to the Board for provisional membership

  2. Review applications for advancement and verify that meaningful proctoring activity has taken place

  3. Review applications for additional proctoring and make a suitable recommendation to the board

V. Proctoring for additional privileges

A. Members of the active, courtesy, or consulting staff who desire additional privileges shall be proctored for such privileges.

B. The department chair shall determine the extent and scope of proctoring. A specific plan for proctoring shall accompany the application for additional privileges to include the name(s) of the proctor(s) and length of time/number and type of cases to be proctored.

FIGURE 4.4

SAMPLE PROCTOR ASSIGNMENT PROCEDURE

Procedure

1. The medical staff office, under direction of the relevant department chair, will assign proctors per rotation of qualified members in the relevant specialty.

2. The medical staff office shall do the following:

   • Send a letter to the provisional practitioner and enclose copies of the appropriate department proctoring/evaluation forms. Label each form "l," "2," etc. Provide a #10 envelope stamped Confidential that's addressed to the medical staff office. Label the envelopes "l," "2," etc. and staple to the appropriately numbered evaluation form. Instruct the new medical staff member of his/her responsibility to attach the form, with patient name and medical record number, on the medical record and to notify his/her proctor.

   • Send a letter and proctoring protocol to the assigned proctor (and alternate), advising him/her to complete the evaluation form (including the patient name and medical record number), place it in the attached envelope, and seal and return it to the medical staff office.

   Note: If the evaluation form is left on the chart—complete or incomplete—and the medical record is due to be returned to the medical records department, the nurse or medical records clerk will be advised to enclose the form in the envelope and return it to the medical staff office.

   • If the proctor does not complete the form, immediately call the provisional practitioner and advise him/her to ask the proctor to review the chart retrospectively.

   • Request that the chart be pulled and made available to the proctor either in medical records or in the medical staff office.

   • When proctors have been assigned and provisional practitioner(s) notified, the medical staff office will assist in physician compliance by performing the following functions:

     — Review daily report on admissions by admitting/attending physician supplied by the medical records/information services department.

     — Compare the report with the listing of provisional practitioners (i.e., medical staff roster). If any provisional practitioner's name appears on the admit list, call his/her office and remind him/her to contact the proctor (give name of proctor and phone number of office) immediately. Remind him/her of his/her responsibility to attach the proctor form(s) to the medical record so that the proctor can complete the form when he/she evaluates the chart. Once the proctor completes the form, he or she should return it to the medical staff office in the envelope provided.

   • As proctor evaluation forms are returned, date stamp and pull the provisional practitioner's credentials file, update the status sheet, and file proctor forms under status sheet. If the case requirement has been met,

FIGURE 4.4   *SAMPLE PROCTOR ASSIGNMENT PROCEDURE (CONT.)*

pull the proctor evaluation forms and status sheet from the file and submit them to the appropriate department chair for review and recommendation.

3. The department chair makes a written recommendation to the credentials committee to advance a practitioner from provisional status, extend the provisional status for a limited period of time, or summarily suspend/terminate the practitioner's privilege(s). The credentials committee makes a recommendation to the medical executive committee to advance a practitioner from provisional status, extend the provisional period for a limited time, or summarily suspend or terminate the practitioner's privilege(s).

Goal: Proctors should complete their proctoring requirements as quickly as possible so that provisional practitioners are eligible for advancement from provisional status versus termination of membership/ privileges.

FIGURE
4.5

INTENDED PRACTICE PLAN

Name: _____

1. I intend to establish (or join) a practice in the following community:_____

2. I will be practicing as a solo /group member practitioner: (circle one)

If practicing with a group, list the name of the group:_____

3. I will admit my patients in need of hospitalization to [hospital name]:
    ❑ Yes   ❑ No

If no, to what institution will you be admit your patients in need of hospitalization? _____

If yes, approximately how many patients per month will you admit? _____

4. I will not be admitting patients; however, I will be referring my patients to [hospital name] when they are in need of acute services.
    ❑ Yes   ❑ No

5. Answer this question only if you perform procedures:
I will perform procedures at [hospital name]. _____
    ❑ Yes   ❑ No

If yes, approximately how many per month? _____

If no, where will you perform procedures? _____

6. I will perform consultations at the request of other physicians at [hospital name].
    ❑ Yes   ❑ No

If no, please provide a brief explanation.
_____

7. I will cross-cover for my partners at [hospital name].
    ❑ Yes   ❑ No

If no, please provide a brief explanation.
_____

8. The following physician has explicitly agreed to provide continuing coverage for my patients when I am not available:_____

FIGURE
4.5
INTENDED PRACTICE PLAN (CONT.)

(Note: As part of your application process, you must submit a statement signed by this physician indicating that he/she explicitly agrees to be available in your absence to provide continuous care to your patients.)

9. I will not use [*hospital name*] for the care of my patients, but desire medical staff appointment to secure participation with various health maintenance or managed care organizations.
   ❑ Yes   ❑ No

10. I agree to treat employees, patients, visitors, and other physicians at [hospital name] in a dignified, professional and courteous manner.
    ❑ Yes   ❑ No

11. I agree to complete my patient records in the timeframes specified and required by the institution.
    ❑ Yes   ❑ No

12. I agree to provide back-up specialty coverage at the request of the medical executive committee.
    ❑ Yes   ❑ No

13. I agree to participate in relevant clinical practice guidelines when such guidelines have been determined by the medical executive committee to influence positively patient outcomes and overall performance.
    ❑ Yes   ❑ No

14. I am/am not employed by any of the following healthcare organizations that have been determined by the board of directors of [*hospital name*] to be in competition with the hospital. (Check one)
    ❑ Am employed   ❑ Am not employed
    [*list of organizations*] _____

15. I own/do not own a significant interest, either personally or corporately, in a healthcare organization that competes with [*hospital name*]. (Check one)
    ❑ Do own   ❑ Do not own

16. I agree/do not agree to establish an office/practice in an area determined to be an area of need by the directors of [*hospital name*]. (Check one)
    ❑ Agree   ❑ Do not agree

I understand that my answers to the above questions will be considered by [*hospital name*] and that appointment, if offered, will be contingent to adherence to this practice plan.

_____ _____   _____
Signature   Date

FIGURE 4.6

SAMPLE BYLAWS LANGUAGE: CATEGORIES OF THE MEDICAL STAFF

SECTION 1: THE ACTIVE CATEGORY

1.1 Qualifications

Appointees to this category must have served on the medical staff for [X] years, be involved in [XX] patient contacts (i.e., a patient contact is defined as an inpatient admission, consultation, outpatient surgical procedure and/or an outpatient ancillary referral) at the [Hospital Name] per [two-year (2)] period, except as expressly waived for practitioners with at least [XX] years of service in the active category or for those physicians who document their efforts to support the hospital's patient care mission to the satisfaction of the MEC and [Board].

In the event that an appointee to the active category does not meet the qualifications for reappointment to the active category, and if the appointee is otherwise abiding by all Bylaws, Rules, Regulations, and policies of the staff, the appointee may be appointed to the affiliate category.

[Note: Bylaws must be tailored to indicate what "involved" means—i.e., admission, surgery, referral, ordering a test or service, etc. It is important for the organization to determine whether its medical staff is going to be "exclusive" or "inclusive".]

1.2 Prerogatives

Appointees to this category may do the following:

1.2.1 Exercise such clinical privileges as are granted by the board
1.2.2 Vote on all matters presented by the medical staff and by the appropriate department and committee of which he or she is a member.
1.2.3 Hold office and sit on or be the chairperson of any committee, unless otherwise specified elsewhere in these bylaws.

1.3 Responsibilities

Appointees to this category may do the following:

1.3.1 Contribute to the organizational and administrative affairs of the medical staff.
1.3.2 Actively participate in recognized functions of the staff appointment including quality/performance improvement, risk management and monitoring activities, including monitoring of new appointees during the provisional period and in discharging other staff functions as may be required.
1.3.3 Fulfill any meeting attendance requirements as established by the medical staff.

SECTION 2. THE AFFILIATE CATEGORY

2.1 Qualifications

The affiliate category is reserved for practitioners who do not meet the eligibility requirements for the active category or who choose not to pursue active status.

2.2 Prerogatives

Appointees to this category may do the following:

2.2.1 Exercise such clinical privileges as are granted by the [Board].

2.2.2 Attend meetings of the staff [and [department/division] of which he or she is an appointee and any staff] or hospital education programs.

2.3 Responsibilities

Appointees to this category must do the following:

2.3.1 Contribute to the organizational and administrative affairs of the medical staff.

2.3.2 Actively participate in recognized functions of the staff appointment including quality/performance improvement, risk management and monitoring activities, including monitoring of new appointees during the provisional period and in discharging other staff functions as may be required.

2.3.3 Fulfill any meeting attendance requirements as established by the medical staff.

SECTION 3. THE HONORARY CATEGORY

The honorary category is restricted to those individuals recommended by the MEC and approved by the board. Appointment to this category is entirely discretionary and may be rescinded at any time. Reappointment to this category is not necessary, as appointees are not eligible for clinical privileges. They may attend medical staff department/division meetings, participate in continuing medical education activities, and may be appointed to committees. They shall not hold office or be eligible to vote.

CASE STUDIES: LOW- AND NO-VOLUME PROVIDERS

The preceding chapters of this book provided a solid understanding of some options available to you when processing membership and privileging requests from a low- or no-volume practitioner. The following case studies and solutions will provide additional insight into the challenges presented by such practitioners.

<table>
<tr><td>CASE STUDY
one</td><td>*The referring physician is not clinically active in the hospital but requests reappointment to the medical staff*</td></tr>
</table>

Gerald Barnes, MD, is a family physician who has been a member of Memorial Medical Center's medical staff for 15 years. Barnes also has an active ambulatory practice. Over the past 15 years, Barnes has routinely admitted and cared for patients at Memorial when they were in need of inpatient services. However, due to recent financial and personal pressures, Barnes has decided to concentrate his medical practice on treating patients in the ambulatory setting.

As a result of this decision, Barnes made arrangements with a hospitalist group to provide inpatient care to his patients. This arrangement, now in its second year, is working well for Barnes, the hospitalists, and the hospital. However, because of the efficiency and reliability of the hospitalists, Barnes has not provided clinical services to hospital patients in more than a year.

Despite the absence of clinical inpatient work, Barnes remains active in the hospital's family medicine department, is a member of the hospital's institutional review board, and continues to serve in a "back-up" capacity in the hospital's emergency department (ED).

Barnes was recently up for reappointment. In accordance with the hospital's bylaws, he submitted a reapplication form to the medical staff office (MSO). His completed reapplication includes a request for "continued privileges in family medicine."

Memorial's medical staff bylaws state that the organization will evaluate privilege requests based on competency data gathered through the hospital's performance improvement program. This requirement hinders Barnes' reappointment because he does not provide inpatient services at Memorial or any other hospital. The department chair does not have access to data that can attest to the practitioner's current

Case study one (cont.)

clinical competence. The chair is therefore concerned that he will be forced to deny Barnes' request for privileges.

In addition, the medical staff bylaws, which were last revised five years ago, indicate that physicians must have at least 24 clinical contacts at the facility within the last two years to qualify for appointment to the active category of the medical staff. Again, Barnes does not meet this requirement.

How would your organization respond to this situation?

Keep in mind the following important facts and concerns when considering how your organization would handle this physician's reappointment request:

- Barnes is a respected member of the community
- There is no evidence insinuating that he is not competent
- He has been on the medical staff for several years and will likely be offended by a "demotion" to the courtesy staff
- If the organization denies Barnes' request for clinical privileges, he will be upset and likely request a fair hearing
- The organization does not have the information needed to satisfy the competency equation

Discussion

Barnes is a fine family practitioner with a good reputation at the hospital and in the community. He has found it more advantageous to provide only ambulatory care but, for a variety of reasons (e.g., collegiality, managed care contracts, prestige, tradition, the possibility that he will once again provide inpatient services), he wishes

Case study one (cont.)

to remain on Memorial's medical staff. Barnes therefore submitted a reappoint-ment application in compliance with the organization's policies and procedures.

Note: The hospital is, in essence, requesting that physicians reapply to the med-ical staff when it sends reapplication and privileging forms to the physician. The MSO ideally should send reapplication forms that are tailored to each physician's medical staff and hospital involvement. Physicians who are not qualified for appointment or privileges should not be given an opportunity to apply or reapply.

Barnes completed the reapplication form exactly as he did in previous years. If the MSO had anticipated this situation, it may have opted to send the physician a form that permitted him only to request privileges to refer and follow.

The MSO must now verify that the physician is qualified for medical staff appointment. This task requires that the MSO query the National Practitioner Data Bank (NPDB), the Office of Inspector General, and the state licensing board. The MSO should then require Barnes to submit one or two letters of recommendation from physicians who can attest to his overall professionalism, dedication to patients, and general competency.

If the department chair knows Barnes well, which is likely, he or she could provide the necessary information as part of his or her recommendation to the credentials committee or medical executive committee (MEC). In addition, it is likely that many MEC members know Barnes and can attest to his general qualifications.

Final disposition of this case

Barnes was reappointed to the active category of the medical staff because of his active support of the hospital's mission. He was assigned to the family practice department with privileges to refer and follow.

CASE STUDY **two**	**The physician is not clinically active in the hospital but seeks medical staff membership and privileges to maintain managed care contracts**

Herbert Roulette, MD, is a plastic surgeon who has been on the medical staff at Glenview Medical Center for 15 years. However, the physician has virtually withdrawn from hospital practice in the last five years and has conducted nearly all his clinical activity in his privately owned plastic surgery center. He is active at the center and participates in a number of managed care contracts with a major insurance company and several self/private pay programs.

Roulette has never been involved significantly in hospital medical staff affairs or in the affairs of the county medical society. Because there is another plastic surgical group in town with a strong affiliation to Glenview, he is not routinely requested to provide plastic surgical consults at the hospitals. Further, because he is on the courtesy staff at Glenview, he does not have ED on-call responsibility.

Every two years, the physician reapplies for medical staff appointment with full plastic surgical clinical privileges. He continues to request these privileges because his contracts with various managed-care organizations require him to maintain medical staff appointment with clinical privileges. These reappointment requests did not pose problems in the past because the hospital's credentialing program was not fully developed.

However, Glenview Medical Center was recently the subject of two corporate negligence suits and its insurance carrier notified the organization that it must make significant improvements to its credentialing policies, procedures, and outcomes. In response, the hospital recently employed, on a part-time basis, a physician director for its credentialing program and charged this individual with the responsibility of seeing to it that appointments, reappointments, and grants of clinical privileges are based on evidence of current clinical competence and adhere to the standards

Case study two (cont.)

detailed in the medical staff bylaws. The credentials program director also organized continuing education for department chairs, credentials committee members, and MEC members that explain their credentialing responsibilities. All medical staff leaders and committee members are now taking these responsibilities more seriously.

In light of these improvements, the department chair is hesitant to forward Roulette's reappointment request to the credentials committee because there is little evidence demonstrating the physician's current clinical competence. Roulette does not work in the hospital, does not perform surgery in conjunction with another physician, and has prohibited the institution access to his office records.

Roulette's attorney recently sent a letter to the credentials committee instructing the organization to process the reappointment application in accordance with the medical staff bylaws and to grant Roulette clinical privileges—unless the credentials committee is able to demonstrate that the physician is incompetent.

The attorney contends that the physician meets all relevant qualifications for both medical staff appointment and clinical privileges. The physician is a board-certified plastic surgeon, has no derogatory information in the NPDB, and is regularly sought out by patients for plastic surgical services.

How would your organization respond to this situation?

Keep in mind the following questions when considering how your organization would handle this physician's reappointment request:

- What steps can you take to gather evidence demonstrating that the physician

Case study two (cont.)

is currently competent to perform plastic surgery?

- What are your threshold criteria for processing requests for privileges to perform plastic surgery?
- How should you react to Roulette's refusal to provide the requested records?
- What value does Roulette add to the medical staff and hospital?
- How should you react to the letter from Roulette's attorney?

Discussion

Roulette's case must be handled carefully. The physician insinuated that he will take legal action if the hospital does not approve his request for medical staff appointment and clinical privileges.

The first step is to send the physician a formal letter to inform him that the MSO will not process his application for clinical privileges until he submits one of the following forms for consideration by the relevant medical staff committee and the board:

1. A report completed by two board-certified plastic surgeons, approved by the hospital, that states that they have conducted a comprehensive review of Roulette's practice. This review should include an analysis of at least 10% of the cases Roulette performed in his office in the last year. The cases must be chosen using a random stratified selection mechanism.

2. Legible photocopies of 10% of his cases for evaluation by a plastic surgeon of the hospital's choosing. The hospital and Roulette should share the expense for the review. The hospital should not ask a plastic surgeon on its medical

staff to conduct this review because of antitrust considerations, even though their review would be acceptable for purposes of determining the quality and necessity of Roulette's practice.

3. A letter from the physician that authorizes an appropriate hospital representative to access and review his office records. Once again, the cost for review of such records should be shared equally by Roulette and the hospital.

The hospital should also inform Roulette that it will only consider his request for reappointment if it receives a completed intended practice plan that indicates how the physician plans to help the hospital and medical staff meet their missions.

The physician should also submit questionnaires that attest to his judgment, skill, overall professional performance, and quality from at least three physicians who regularly interact with his patients as either referring or treating physicians.

Final disposition of this case

The hospital did not process Roulette's application for reappointment and clinical privileges because the physician failed to provide information necessary for the hospital to assess his competency.

The physician and his attorney did not respond to letters sent by the MSO that quoted the medical staff bylaws in regard to the "burden on the physician" and "the need for inactive practitioners to state their intention regarding their support of the hospital's mission."

| CASE STUDY | The provider treats the majority or all of |
| *three* | his or her patients at another facility |

Patricia Smith, MD, is a general surgeon who specializes in laparoscopic surgery. Smith has been practicing in Youngsville for seven years, and Memorial Medical Center is her primary hospital. She is the laparoscopic program director at Memorial and she is compensated for assuming this leadership position.

Smith also maintains courtesy appointment at St. Mary's Hospital and has full clinical privileges in general surgery, including advanced laparoscopic work. However, the physician does not take ED back-up call at St. Mary's and is absent from nearly all general staff, committee, and department meetings. Despite these shortcomings, no one on staff at St. Mary's or Memorial doubts Smith's clinical qualifications.

Smith recently submitted her reappointment application for medical staff membership at St. Mary's. She is once again requesting full clinical privileges. The MSO at St. Mary's learned that Smith is clinically active at Memorial and that she is not subject to any investigation, disciplinary action, or other troubling activity. In addition, the department chair at Memorial has reported that Smith is clinically competent to perform all requested privileges.

However, the general surgery department chair at St. Mary's—William Jones, MD— is concerned about Smith's lack of clinical activity at the facility. Jones is also concerned that Smith may be ineligible for reappointment at St. Mary's because she is the compensated director of the laparoscopic program at Memorial and therefore in potential conflict with St. Mary's. Unfortunately, St. Mary's medical staff bylaws and board policies do not address potential physician conflicts of interest.

The department chair has questioned Smith's qualifications for medical staff reappointment because of her lack of clinical activity, lack of support of the ED, and lack

Case study three (cont.)

of participation in medical staff activities. However, the credentials committee has proceeded to fairly and objectively process Smith's reappointment application and concluded that she is qualified for the clinical privileges.

The credentials committee based this decision on the excellent work Smith performs at Memorial. The committee then reviewed its medical staff bylaws to determine whether there are any grounds on which to deny Smith's request for reappointment to the courtesy staff.

How would your organization respond to this situation?

Keep in mind the following questions and facts when considering how your organization would handle this physician's reappointment request:

- Does your medical staff and hospital have a policy addressing potential conflicts of interest?
- In the absence of a board policy on this issue, are there grounds for denying Smith's request for reappointment?
- Smith is not a no- or low-volume practitioner. She has a significant clinical practice at another inpatient facility.

Discussion

Smith is a well-qualified physician. It would not be difficult for St. Mary's to determine that she is indeed qualified for reappointment and requested privileges. However, the physician and Memorial Hospital must be willing to provide St. Mary's with all requested volume and performance data in a timely manner.

Case study three (cont.)

Final disposition of this case

St. Mary's asked Smith to complete an intended practice plan. The board then approved the plan and agreed that similar action should be taken in the future when processing an application from a low- and no-volume provider.

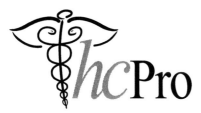

RELATED PRODUCTS FROM *HCPRO*

Books

How to Recruit and Develop Physician Leaders: A Strategy for Medical Staff Leadership Development

By Albert L. Fritz, MHA, Todd Sagin, MD, JD, and Richard A. Sheff, MD

The success of your organization is, to a large extent, dependent upon the success of your medical staff. Strong, effective physician leadership is critical for achieving a truly effective medical staff. You need to invest in leadership development and plan for leadership succession.

That's why we've developed the modern solution to your medical staff leadership challenge. This book will guide you through the steps of how to identify, recruit, and retain successful leaders for an effective medical staff. You'll learn, step-by-step, how to

- Clarify the leadership role with job descriptions
- Recruit physician leaders
- Ensure you have a sound nomination and selection process
- Train your physician leaders
- Implement a succession plan

10 Steps to Successful Physician Profiling

By Robert Marder, MD, and Richard A. Sheff, MD

Physician profiling to assess physicians' competence is essential in the reappointment process. But more important than simply reappointing physicians, you need to provide meaningful feedback to help them improve their quality of care.

To do that, you must decide what data to collect, how to collect it, and how to communicate your results to help physicians improve performance.

Save time, money, and resources

This how-to guide outlines a 10-step comprehensive profiling process that will help you create a solid physician performance feedback system. You'll learn how to collect meaningful data, evaluate it using predetermined benchmarks, and communicate your findings to initiate physician performance improvement.

Stop wasting time—give physicians relevant feedback so they can act

You'll also receive a customizable physician performance report. You'll learn how to consolidate your collected data—from clinical quality, service quality, and activity to resource utilization and even peer relationships—and display results so physicians can easily see where they need to improve. With pre-calculated formulas, you'll be able recognize performance trends and show physicians where they rank in comparison to their peers. You can also tailor the report to track and measure physician behavior patterns in your facility.

The Top 30 Medical Staff Policies and Procedures, Third Edition

By Hugh Greeley, Richard A. Sheff, MD, and ALbert L. Fritz, MHA
You need to ensure that your medical staff office policies and procedures are clear, concise, and compliant with the 2004 JCAHO standards. Save time—we've done the work for you!

The Top 30 Medical Staff Policies and Procedures, Third Edition, is a hands-on tool that will provide you with 30 sample policies and procedures for the most complex, challenging medical staff topics. Plus, you'll receive each policy in both print format and on a companion CD-ROM that makes customization quick and easy.

Updated to Reflect the 2004 JCAHO Standards

We've updated the policies and procedures—including peer review, medical staff leadership selection, and telemedicine—to reflect the 2004 JCAHO standards. Plus, you'll receive five new critical policies and procedures that have become increasingly important to medical staffs all across the country.

Core Privileges: A Practical Approach to Development and Implementation, Second Edition

By Hugh P. Greeley, Laura Harrington, RN, CPHQ, Beverly E. Pybus, CPMSM, and Richard A. Sheff, MD
Medical staff privileging continues to be an ongoing challenge for medical staff services professionals as you try to meet JCAHO standards and ensure the provision of quality care. This

comprehensive manual provides you with step-by-step guidelines and tools to develop and implement the most efficient and consistent privileging system available: the core privileging approach.

We've done the work for you! **Core Privileges, Second Edition** makes your job easier by providing dozens of sample policies, procedures, and privileging forms to guide the implementation of your own core privileging system. You'll receive approximately 20 new procedures and new subspecialties, including trauma surgery, surgical oncology, pediatric anesthesiology, and more.

Newsletters

Would you like to review any of the following newsletters? Call us at 800/650-6787 and we will forward a complimentary copy of each to your attention.

Medical Staff Briefing

Medical Staff Briefing supports medical staff leaders and MSSPs by providing up-to-the-minute information, time-saving tools, and expert advice—ensuring compliance with government and accreditor regulations, high quality care, and improved relationships at all levels. Every issue is filled with new ideas and crucial information you need to do your job better. As a subscriber, you could receive information such as:

- Proven STRATEGIES for developing effective physician performance feedback reports
- Expert ADVICE on how to privilege and reappoint low volume providers
- TIPS to comply with JCAHO's 2004 medical staff standards
- Field-tested IDEAS to recruit and train physicians for leadership roles
- New APPROACHES for dealing with disruptive or impaired physicians
- GUIDELINES to help you develop privileging criteria for new technologies

The Credentialing Resource Center (CRC)

From credentialing AHPs to completing core privileges for each of your departments and physician profiling, how are you fitting in your traditional credentialing and privileging duties?

Many of you have told us that you are having a tough time juggling new concerns and responsibilities while performing the day-to-day tasks of running a medical staff office. The **Credentialing Resource Center** provides you with the step-by-step advice, tools, and proven best practices from both credentialing experts working in the field and your peers. and proven tools that you need to make your job a whole lot easier.

As a member of the **Credentialing Resource Center,** you'll receive the following exclusive members-only benefits:

- *Clinical Privilege White Papers*—These documents offer privileging criteria on brand-new, controversial, or difficult areas or procedures—check out the free White Paper enclosed
- **Fax/Email Express**—When news happens that just can't wait, subscribers receive late-breaking information via fax or e-mail to keep them informed on the latest credentialing news
- **E-mail Chat Group**—Network with over 200 other medical staff services professionals on Medical Staff Talk and get answers to your credentialing questions instantly
- **Special Reports**—Whenever new regulations are enacted that require your immediate attention, we'll publish an independent Special Report and send it your way
- **Credentialing Solutions**—This reoccurring column gives you answers and advice to all of your credentialing questions and concerns
- *Managed Care Credentialing*—A supplement to **Briefings on Credentialing** on how to credential practitioners in the manage care environment
- **Survey Review**—Recently surveyed facilities share in this tri-monthly article what JCAHO surveyors focused on, as well as offer survival tips to help other facilities prepare for their own surveys
- **CE quizzes**—Every three months, you'll receive a CE quiz for a chance to earn continuing education units toward your NAMSS certification

---

To obtain additional information, to order any of the above products, or to comment on *A Practical Guide to Assessing the Competency of Low-Volume Providers,* please contact us at:

Mail:	**Toll-free telephone:** 800/650-6787
HCPro	**Toll-free fax:** 800/639-8511
P.O. Box 1168	**E-mail:** *customerservice@hcpro.com*
Marblehead, MA 01945	**Internet:** *www.hcmarketplace.com*
